PROTEIN BIOCHEMISTRY, SYNTHESIS, STRUCTURE AND CELLULAR FUNCTIONS

SERUM ALBUMIN

STRUCTURE, FUNCTIONS AND HEALTH IMPACT

PROTEIN BIOCHEMISTRY, SYNTHESIS, STRUCTURE AND CELLULAR FUNCTIONS

Additional books in this series can be found on Nova's website under the Series tab.

Additional E-books in this series can be found on Nova's website under the E-book tab.

PROTEIN BIOCHEMISTRY, SYNTHESIS, STRUCTURE AND CELLULAR FUNCTIONS

SERUM ALBUMIN

STRUCTURE, FUNCTIONS AND HEALTH IMPACT

ROBERT J. ALEKSEEV
AND
ALISA L. REBANE
EDITORS

Nova Science Publishers, Inc.
New York

For permission to use material from this book please contact us:
Telephone 631-231-7269; Fax 631-231-8175
Web Site: http://www.novapublishers.com

Library of Congress Cataloging-in-Publication Data

Serum albumin : structure, functions, and health impact / editors, Robert J. Alekseev and Alisa L. Rebane.
p. ; cm.
Includes bibliographical references and index.
ISBN 978-1-62100-231-4 (hardcover)
I. Alekseev, Robert J. II. Rebane, Alisa L.
[DNLM: 1. Serum Albumin--physiology. 2. Serum Albumin--chemistry. 3. Serum Albumin--metabolism. WH 400]
LC classification not assigned
572'.6--dc23

2011032417

Published by Nova Science Publishers, Inc. †New York

CONTENTS

PREFACE

Serum albumin is the most abundant plasma protein in mammals. Albumin is essential for maintaining the osmotic pressure needed for proper distribution of body fluids between intravascular compartments and body tissues. It also acts as a plasma carrier by non-specifically binding several hydrophobic steroid hormones and as a transport protein for hemin and fatty acids. This book presents current research in the study of the structure, functions and health impacts of serum albumin. Topics include the catalytic activities of serum albumin; the interaction of serum albumin with anesthetics; microparticulate drug delivery systems based on serum albumin; hydration of human serum albumin and extracting physical properties of serum albumin using osmotic pressure.

Chapter 1 – Serum albumin is a multi-functional protein with unique ligand-binding capabilities. In addition, it possesses a number of catalytic activities. The ligand-binding function of serum albumin has been profoundly studied and reported by protein chemists, cell biologists, nutritionists, pharmacologists, and clinicians. Therefore, in this chapter, the authors will only touch upon this important albumin's function and concentrate on discussing the mechanisms and biological significance of albumin's catalytic polyfunctionality. At the same time, information about the structural organization of serum albumin is provided in the first part of the chapter. It will help to shed light on the unique ligand-binding capabilities of the protein and can provide a structural basis for the discussion of its enzymatic properties. In the second section of the chapter, they will list all reported catalytic activities of albumin and describe mechanisms of these activities, if known.

Chapter 2 – The molecular mechanism of anesthesia is one of the long-standing unresolved problems in medical science. Although two representative theories of anesthesia, a protein receptor theory based on the direct binding of anesthetics to several signal receptor proteins in nerve membranes and a lipid membrane theory based on the indirect binding of anesthetics to nerve membranes with high content of lipids, have been argued up to now, the action mechanism has not yet been clarified. More recently, the emphasis has shifted from theories oflipid perturbation to the idea that anesthetics bind directly to specific proteins.Serum albumin is an abundant plasma protein transporting a wide variety of drugs and endogenous compounds and has been widely used for life-science studies. A number of studies on the binding of such drugs and compounds to serum albumin have been reported since pioneer works by Foster et al. in late 1950s. In the beginning of 1990s, Carter et al. determined the detailed molecular structure of serum albumin from the X-ray structural analysis, and subsequently the binding sites of several small ligands for serum albumin were identified on the structure. In such circumstances, serum albumin has been regarded a good model for anesthetic action, and the binding data of anesthetics to serum albumin examined by various physicochemical methods have been accumulated for the last several decades. Most of the binding studies of anesthetics to serum albumin showed that there exist weak but specific interactions between serum albumin and anesthetics, and crystallographic data suggested that all anesthetics bind fatty-acid binding sites on serum albumin without binding the unique site to each anesthetic. On the other hand, a comparative study of ligand interactions indicated that the binding mode of anesthetics is pronouncedly different from that of specific binders such as fatty acids. Here model studies of anesthetic action by using serum albumin are reviewed, and characteristic binding modes of anesthetics to serum albumin are elucidated in connection with the anesthetic mechanism.

Chapter 3 – Drug delivery systems are developed to improve the efficacy, bioavailability and pharmacokinetic properties of therapeutically active molecules. These systems have to meet precise requirements, like biocompatibility and biodegradability. Furthermore, the active molecule has to be bound and protected by the system until it reaches a physiological target, and then the system is able to release the molecule in a controlled manner. The release kinetics of the bioactive molecule by an ideal delivery system is designed for an optimized therapeutic effect in vivo, and this kinetics is synchronized with the degradation kinetics of the system itself. Microparticulate drug delivery systems, i.e. microcapsules and microspheres, present an interesting surface-to-volume ratio, favoring exchange phenomena between their load and the physiological environment after administration. The interactions and release kinetics of various molecules with microparticles can be precisely controlled by the size of the particles, and by the parameters of the process used to produce them. Many methods are now developed to produce microparticles, based on physical, physico-chemical or chemical processes. Easily available and often biocompatible, biopolymers play an increasing role among the materials available to constitute the frame of microparticles. In this context, serum albumin is an emerging biopolymer presenting very attractive properties for its use as a constitutive material for microparticulate drug delivery systems. This endogeneous macromolecule, already used in human health for the treatment of various diseases by different routes, is perfectly biocompatible and biodegradable. Albumin is known for its binding properties towards various xenobiotics, and for its solubilizing properties towards hydrophobic compounds. Moreover, albumin presents physicochemical properties like high solubility in water, low viscosity in solution, interfacial properties, denaturation upon heating, which can be very useful in encapsulation processes. Furthermore, this protein bears many functional groups available for chemical modifications needed for encapsulation by chemical methods.

This paper reviews the methods used to produce microparticles from serum albumin for drug delivery purposes. The methods based on physical, physico-chemical and chemical processes will be described, as well as studies dealing with the properties of the resulting microparticles.

Chapter 4 – This work describes the basic principles of a novel experimental approach for studying the hydration of proteins. This method, based on the calorimetric measurements, allows for the simultaneous monitoring of the excess partial enthalpies of water and the protein obtained in the entire range of water contents. Human serum albumin (HSA) was used as a model protein. The excess partial quantities of water and HSA are very sensitive to the hydration level. At the lowest water contents, HSA is in a rigid (glassy) state. Changes of the excess thermochemical function can mainly be attributed to water addition. A transition from the glassy to the flexible state of HSA is accompanied by significant changes in the excess partial quantities of water and HSA. This transition appears at water weight fraction (w_1) of 0.06 when charged and polar groups of HSA are covered. Excess partial quantities reach their fully hydrated values at $w_1 > 0.4$ when coverage of both polar and weakly interacting surface elements is complete. At the highest water contents, water addition has no significant effect on the excess thermochemical function. At $w_1 > 0.4$, the observed changes in the excess function can solely be attributed to changes in the protein structure.

Chapter 5 – The tryptophan fluorescence of human serum albumin (HSA) at addition of ionic surfactants (anionic surfactant sodium dodecyl sulfate SDS and cationic surfactant cethyltrimethylammonium bromide CTAB) in protein solution at various values of pH was investigated, what gave information about mechanism of denaturation of HSA under action of ionic surfactants. The analysis of non-polarized and polarized steady-state tryptophan fluorescence of HSA in solutions with SDS and CTAB was done. The experimental dependences of intensity and polarization of tryptophan fluorescence of HSA on concentrations of SDS (0 – 7 mM) and CTAB (0 – 7 mM) in solutions at various values of pH (3.5 – 8.0) were found out. The quenching of tryptophan fluorescence of HSA in solutions with ionic surfactants was registered, and the value of this quenching depends not only on concentration of surfactant, but also on value of pH. The polarization of tryptophan fluorescence of HSA in solutions with ionic surfactants increases. The calculation of parameters of rotational diffusion (coefficient of rotational diffusion, time of rotational relaxation and effective Einstein's radius) of HSA molecules in solutions with various concentrations of SDS and CTAB at various values of pH was done. In solutions with ionic surfactants SDS and CTAB the decrease of coefficient of rotational diffusion of HSA, the increase of time of rotational relaxation of HSA, corresponding to disordering owing to thermal diffusion, and the increase of effective Einstein's radius of HSA molecules take place, what speaks about denaturation of HSA under action of these ionic surfactants – decondensation of protein globules with increase of its linear-longitude sizes and unfolding of amino-acidic chain of protein. On basis of received dependences the conclusion was done, that denaturation of HSA under action of cationic surfactant CTAB has one-stage character at all investigated values of pH, but denaturation of HSA under action of anionic surfactant SDS has more complex character – at values of pH, lower than pI of HSA, denaturation has two stage-character, and at values of pH, higher than pI of HSA, denaturation has one-stage character. It is shown that more deep denaturation of HSA under action of CTAB takes place at values of pH, higher than pI of HSA, on contrary more deep denaturation of HSA under action of SDS takes place at values of pH, lower than pI of HSA.

Chapter 6 – Albumin is the most abundant protein in human plasma, being present at a concentration of 30-50 g/l. It has several important functions in the blood including assistance in maintaining osmotic pressure; transport of hormones (in particular fat soluble ones); transportation of fatty acids to the liver; transportation of drugs; and maintenance of pH. It has a long plasma half life – typically 20 days (Peters 1996). This combination of low biological activity, long half life and ability to bind fatty (and therefore poorly aqueous soluble) molecules makes albumin an attractive candidate for incorporation into drug delivery/formulation systems and its use in this role has been examined over the last twenty years (Peters 1996). More recently there has also been a growing awareness that albumin may, under certain circumstances, be selectively accumulated by solid tumours (Clorius et al,

1995; Goldshaid et al; 2010). Clearly this accumulation of albumin offers the potential for improved delivery of drugs to specific sites of action, particularly to tumours. The search for effective drug delivery systems is one of the major challenges facing pharmaceutical research, especially for biomedically important molecules such as proteins, peptide-based vaccines, tumour therapeutic agents, antimicrobials and lipodrugs. A procedure has been developed whereby human serum albumin (HSA) can be use as a delivery vehicle for a number of these biological molecules by exploiting its physiological role as the bodies' main fatty acid carrier. Using essentially fatty acid free HSA (HSAff) it is possible to form stable complexes with compounds that contain alkyl chains (called lipo-compounds). Two lipo-compounds have been used to develop this system, a novel antimicrobial peptide and the neurotransmitter γ-amino-n-butyric acid GABA conjugated with C8 or C14 alkyl chains (Hussain and Siligardi 2006, 2010). Both lipo-compounds were evaluated confirming that the formation of HSA-lipo compound complexes had a mutual stabilizing effect on both HSAff and lipo-compounds. The protease enzymes pronase was used to show that the alkyl chains of the lipo-compounds bound to HSAff conferred a similar if not greater resistance to enzymatic degradation than the HSA for clinical use such as Baxter Albumin and Zenalbumin, which contain sodium caprylate and acetyl tryptophanate. Here the authors indicated that the use of HSAff as a carrier for lipidated drugs might confer higher biostability to the lipidated drugs providing a novel formulation method for therapeutic use. The increased stability of the lipo-compounds when formulated using the HSAff was not observed when HSA containing fatty acid (HSAfa) was used (Hussain and Siligardi 2006 and 2010). Furthermore in the case of the antimicrobial lipopeptide there was an increased in activity with the HSAff formulation suggesting that besides conferring stability it also enhanced bioavailability of compounds that would otherwise exist as insoluble micelles in aqueous media. These findings have allowed them to develop a simple and effective way of delivering lipo containing compounds using fatty acid free HSA as the drug carrier.

Chapter 7 – The relation between several pathological diseases (Alzheimer, BSE, Creutzfeldt-Jacob disease, etc.) and the formation of proteinaceous deposits in plaques, amyloid fibrils and filaments has led a great deal of renewed attention to the topic of protein aggregation. Different factors such as pH, temperature, solvents, protein concentration, cosolutes, etc., modulate the aggregation process. In particular, the presence of metal ions can modify inter- or intra-molecular interaction thus exerting different effects on proteins stability. In the present chapter the authors show that the addition of exogenous ions to a solution of partially denaturated Bovine Serum Albumin (BSA) promotes molecular aggregation and gel formation (cold gelation). On the other hand, they describe how BSA native structure is stabilized by the presence of endogenous ions, which are so strongly bound that can be separated by HPLC treatment only.

In: Serum Albumin: Structure, Functions and Health Impact ISBN: 978-1-62100-231-4
Editors: R. J. Alekseev and A. L. Rebane

Chapter 1

CATALYTIC ACTIVITIES OF SERUM ALBUMIN: MECHANISMS, BIOLOGICAL FUNCTION AND PRACTICAL APPLICATIONS

Tatyana S. Godovikova,[1,2] Yulia V. Gerasimova[1,*] and Dmitry G. Knorre[1]

[1]Institute of Chemical Biology and Fundamental Medicine, Siberian Branch of Russian Academy of Sciences, Novosibirsk, Russia

[2]Novosibirsk State University, Novosibirsk, Russia

Serum albumin is a multi-functional protein with unique ligand-binding capabilities. In addition, it possesses a number of catalytic activities. The ligand-binding function of serum albumin has been profoundly studied and reported by protein chemists, cell biologists, nutritionists, pharmacologists, and clinicians. Therefore, in this chapter, we will only touch upon this important albumin's function and concentrate on discussing the mechanisms and biological significance of albumin's catalytic polyfunctionality. At the same time, information about the structural organization of serum albumin is provided in the first part of the chapter. It will help to shed light on the unique ligand-binding capabilities of the protein and can provide a structural basis for the discussion of its enzymatic properties. In the second section of the chapter, we will list all reported catalytic activities of albumin and describe mechanisms of these activities, if known.

In addition, we will report how albumin's modifications by endogenous and exogenous compounds affect its catalytic properties. Finally, we will dwell upon possible applications of the catalytic activities of this protein in medical practice and life science research. For instance, the wide range of reactions catalyzed by albumin, together with its natural abundance and relatively high catalytic efficiency at extreme temperatures, make the protein an appealing catalyst for biotechnological applications, including bioprocesses in non-aqueous solvents. Another possible application of the protein is detoxification of harmful substances at low substrate concentrations.

[*]Present address: Chemistry Department, University of Central Florida, 4000 Central Florida Blvd., Orlando, FL 32816, USA

1. STRUCTURE OF SERUM ALBUMIN

Serum albumin is a single-chain protein synthesized in and secreted from liver cells. Many researchers have studied the structure of serum albumin, its properties and functions to understand the protein's interactions with a number of ligands (Peters, 1996; Kragh-Hansen *et al.*, 2002). Nowadays, the primary sequences of serum albumins from several species, including human (Behrens *et al.*, 1975), cow (Brown, 1975), rat (Strauss *et al.,* 1977), sheep (Brown *et al.,* 1989), horse (Ho *et al.,* 1993), frog (Moskaitis *et al.,* 1989) and salmon (Byrnes and Gannon, 1990), are known. There is 70-80% of homology of amino acid sequences within mammal serum albumins (Peters, 1996). In particular, human serum albumin (HSA) and bovine serum albumin (BSA) share a sequence homology of 76% (Huang *et al.*, 2004). Being homologous proteins, BSA and HSA have very similar biological functions. Since the catalytic activities of human and bovine serum albumins are the most studied, the description of albumins' three-dimensional structure will be limited to these two proteins.

The human protein is comprised of 585 amino acids and has a molecular mass of 66.5 kDa. Its amino acid sequence is characterized by a large percentage of cysteine residues (6%). These residues, except one, are involved in 17 disulfide bonds, which are important in stabilizing the HSA structure. HSA also contains a large number of charged amino acids (31%). Curiously, there is only one tryptophan residue in the protein. The three-dimensional structure of HSA remained largely unknown until the first crystal structure of HSA at 2.8 Å resolution was reported in 1992 (He and Carter, 1992). Since then, several independent X-ray structural determinations of HSA have been published (Sugio *et al.* 1999; Curry *et al.*, 1998). According to the data of X-ray analysis, the HSA isolated from blood, as well as its recombinant version (rHSA), is a heart-shaped molecule 80 Å on a side, with an average thickness of 30 Å (see Figure 1). It has a high α-helical content (67%). The tertiary structure of HSA is composed of three repeating domains: domain I (residues 1-195), domain II (residues 196-383), and domain III (residues 384-585), which are characterized by a common motif of 10 α-helices (Sugio *et al.* 1999). Each domain is divided into two subdomains (A, B) where the helices h1-h4 in subdomain A are homologous to h7-h10 in subdomain B. The partially overlapping regions of the domains are a consequence of the helical continuation from the C-terminal portion of the IB and IIB helices to the N-terminal helices of IIA and IIIA (helices: $h10_{I}$-$h1_{II}$ and $h10_{II}$-$h1_{III}$), respectively (Dockal *et al.*, 1999).

Based on the results of combined phosphorescence depolarization-hydrodynamic modeling study (Ferrer *et al*, 2001), the overall conformation of HSA in neutral solution was proposed to be very similar to that observed in the crystal form.

The domain II and III of HSA contain two primary drug binding sites, known as Sudlow's site I and site II (Sudlow *et al.*, 1975). Several additional sites were also observed (Bhattacharya *et al.*, 2000; Ghuman *et al.*, 2005; Lejon *et al.*, 2004; Petitpas *et al.*, 2003). Crystallographic structural analysis of HSA-ligand complexes provides a structural basis to understand HSA's role in drugs metabolism (Ghuman *et al.*, 2005; Yang *et al.*, 2007).

Bovine serum albumin, according to Brown (Brown, 1975), is composed of 582 amino acid residues. The later study by Hirayama *et. al.* (Hirayama *et. al.* 1990) corrected that the primary sequence of bovine protein contains 583 amino acid residues. BSA contains a single cysteine and eight pairs of disulfide bonds arranged in a way similar to those of HSA (He and Carter, 1992).

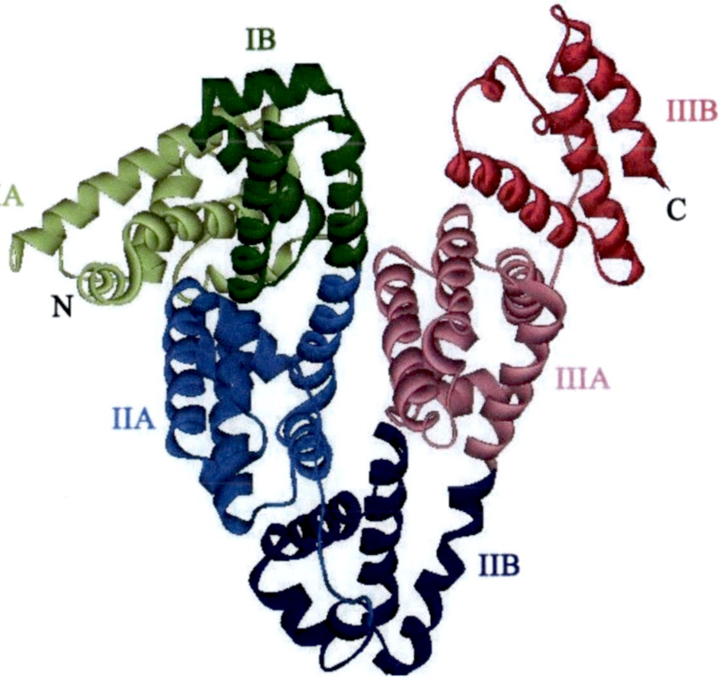

Figure 1.Three-dimensional structure of HSA (based on the structure obtained by Sugio *et al*, 1999, PDB ID 1AO6).

Despite 76% of amino acid sequence homologybetween HSA and BSA, the three-dimensional structure of the bovine protein has not been determined so far. According to the amino acid sequence proposed by Brown, the structural features of BSA are similar to those of HSA. Like its human analog, bovine serum albumin is composed of three homologous domains (I, II and III), each of which is subdivided into two subdomains. The domains contain the following structure: large double loop - short connecting segment-small double loop - long connecting segment-large double loop - interdomainal connecting segment (Brown, 1976). The helical segments in each domain are homological to those of HSA. However, the data from chemical cross-linking experiments obtained by Huang *et. al.* (Huang *et al*, 2004) suggests that there are some structural differences between BSA and HSA in domain II. BSA contains a high content of Asp, Glu, Ala, Leu and Lys residues, which is similar to HSA.

2. Catalytic Activities of Serum Albumin: Mechanisms and Biological Function

Serum albumin is traditionally considered an inert protein, which mainly participates in sustaining the blood pH and osmotic pressure and serves as a carrier and transporter for a number of ligands. However, a large volume of data accumulated so far argues that the protein possesses various catalytic activities. Reactions found to be catalyzed by serum albumin can be divided into four groups: 1) hydrolytic reactions resulting in a cleavage of different bonds (hydrolase activity); 2) double bond formation (lyase activity); 3) reactions of isomerization (isomerase activity); 4) oxidative-reductive transformations (thiol peroxidase activity).

2.1. Albumin as a Hydrolase

2.1.1. RNA-Hydrolyzing Activity of Serum Albumin

Recently (Takahashi *et al.*, 2006), it has been found that bovine serum albumin (BSA) possesses RNase-like activity. The efficiency of BSA-catalyzed RNA cleavage was shown to be concentration-dependent. The cleavage products contained 2',3'-cyclophosphate and 5'-hydroxyl groups (Takahashi *et al.*, 2006). The observed activity was inhibited by acetylation of the protein, which allowed the authors to suggest that RNA degradation in the presence of the protein might be regulated by the positive charge of its lysine residues. Later, Gerasimova and colleagues have shown that similar but significantly higher activity is inherent to human serum albumin (HSA) (Gerasimova *et al.*, 2008a; Gerasimova *et al.*, 2008b; Gerasimova *et al.*, 2010). The cleavage of phosphodiester bonds in several RNA substrates was catalyzed by both the protein isolated from blood and its recombinant analogue (rHSA). When compared with RNase-like activity of BSA, HSA turned out to be one order of magnitude more efficient in RNA hydrolysis than its bovine analog (rate constants for RNA hydrolysis were calculated to be $0.028 \pm 0.0006\ min^{-1}$ and $0.0033 \pm 0.0003\ min^{-1}$ for HSA and BSA, respectively).

Authors (Gerasimova *et al.*, 2010) revealed that RNA hydrolysis in the presence of HSA and rHSA proceeded via 2',3'-cyclophosphate intermediates in accordance with acid-base mechanism of catalysis (Scheme 1). The classic bell-shaped pH profile for HSA-catalyzed RNA hydrolysis can reflect the participation of two protein's ionogenic groups in the catalysis. The pH optimum for RNA-hydrolyzing activity of HSA was found to be 5.5. It was close to the optimal conditions for RNase T1 (Osterman and Walz, 1978), which has a histidine and a glutamate residue important for the catalysis, but was acid-shifted in comparison with the optimal values for pancreatic RNase A (Herries *et al.*, 1962) or human RNase 1 (delCardayre and Raines, 1995), which have catalytic histidine residues. However, since the ionization constant values for the protein amino acid functional groups highly depend on the protein's microenvironment, the obtained data did not allow the authors to unambiguously determine the amino acid residues of albumin involved in the catalysis of RNA cleavage.

Although HSA hydrolyzed RNA in a sequence-independent manner, the major cleavage of the substrates used occurred within the U-A and C-A sequences (Gerasimova *et al.*, 2010). The same specificity of RNA cleavage was observed for BSA by Takahashi and colleagues (Takahashi *et al.*, 2006). The efficacy of HSA-catalyzed hydrolysis of phosphodiester bonds in homopolyribonucleotides depended on the type of the substrate (Gerasimova *et al.*, 2010). Albumin was shown to be the most efficient in the hydrolysis of poly(C) substrate, which is analogous to the specificity displayed by RNase A and human RNase 1 (Table 1). However, the catalytic efficacy of HSA towards poly(A) was found to be only twice as low as towards poly(U) substrate (Gerasimova *et al.*, 2010).

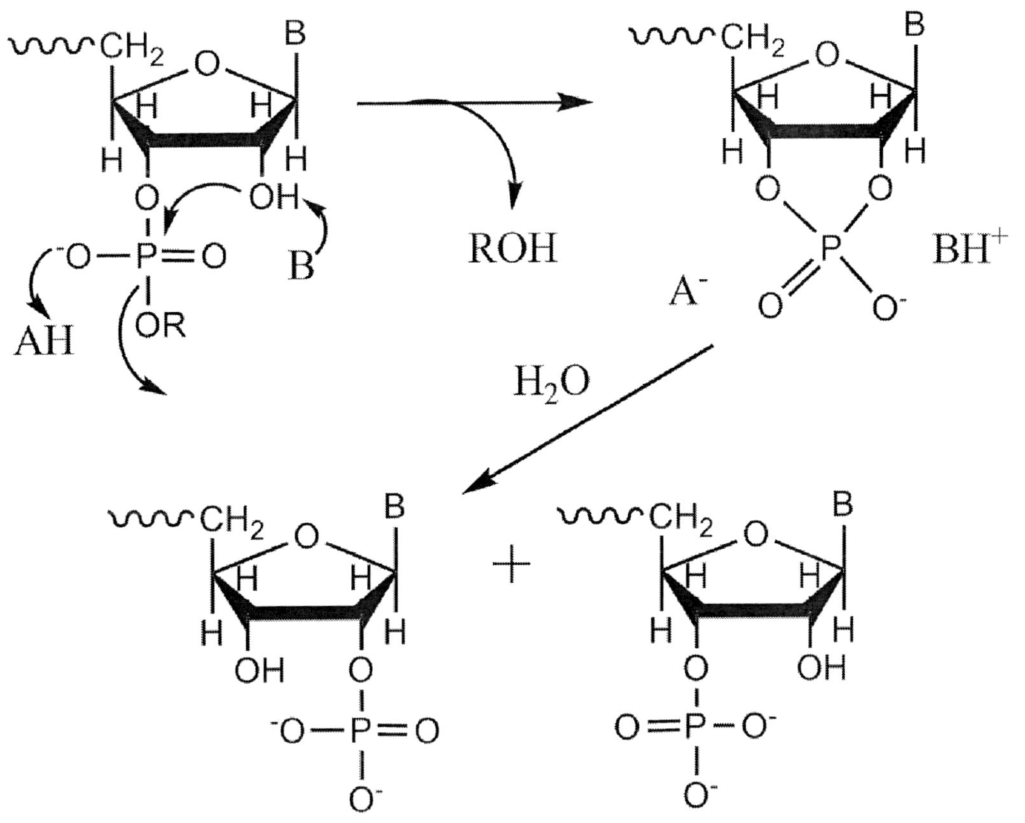

Scheme 1.

Table 1. Relative activity of RNase A, human RNases and HAS for polyribonucleotide hydrolysis [a]

Protein	poly(C)	poly(U)	poly(A)
RNase A[b]	100 %	4.7 %	0.005 %
Human RNase 1[c]	100 %	3.5 %	0.03 %
Human RNases 2 and 3[c]	100 %	1240 %	0 %
HSA	100 %	2.2 %	0.9 %

[a]The activity of each protein in the reaction of poly(U) and poly(A) hydrolysis was calculated taking the activity for poly(C) hydrolysis as 100 %.

[b] According to delCardayre and Raines, 1995. [c] According to Sorrentino and Libonati, 1994.

Taken together, the data on specificity and pH dependence of HSA-catalyzed RNA hydrolysis distinguish albumin from the secretory human ribonucleases. Similar efficacy and cleavage pattern for natural albumin preparation and the recombinant protein can serve as an additional criterion to prove the intrinsic RNA-cleaving property of albumin.

Although albumin's activity in RNA hydrolysis is low in comparison with ribonucleases, the possibility that HSA can participate in extracellular RNAs degradation cannot be excluded, since the concentration of albumin in human blood is rather high (about 0.6 mM) (Peters, 1996). The discovered activity of HSA may have an important biological role. For instance, RNA-cleavage activity of albumin may act as a defense mechanism against circulating nucleic acid from other (i.e., pathogenic) organisms. Modification of lysine residues (non-enzymatic glycation, *N*-homocysteinylation, and *N*-phosphorylation) suppressed albumin-mediated hydrolysis of RNA (Gerasimova *et al.*, 2008a; Gerasimova *et al.*, 2008b). The inhibitory effect of albumin's modification on its RNA-hydrolyzing activity may have an important physiological consequence. For example, the elevated level of lysine-directed HSA modifications may lead to the increased level of extracellular nucleic acids. Another hypothesis is that albumin may participate in the metabolism of endogenous extracellular RNA. From the pharmaceutical point of view, the RNA-cleaving activity of HSA should be taking into account while designing therapeutic siRNA. Albumin, along with other blood RNases, can cleave siRNAs, thus reducing their therapeutic effect.

2.1.2. Pseudo-Esterase Activity of Serum Albumin

The esterase activity of albumin has been known for over 60 years. In particular, the hydrolysis of *p*-nitrophenol esters by HSA was first reported in 1951 (Dirsk and Boyer, 1951). Since then, serum albumin has been reported to catalyze the hydrolysis of a number of substances, including alpha-naphthyl acetate, phenyl acetate, 1-naphthyl *N*-methylcarbamate (Casida and Augustinsson, 1959a), long- and short-chain fatty acid esters (Tove, 1962), *p*-nitrophenyl acetate (Tildon and Ogilvie, 1972; Means and Bender, 1975), beta-naphthyl acetate (Morikawa *et al.*, 1979), aspirin (Rainsford *et al.*, 1980), cyclophosphamide (Kwon *et al.*, 1987), ketoprofen glucuronide (Dubois-Presle *et al.*, 1995), nicotinate esters (Salvi *et al.*, 1997), organophosphorus pesticides (Sogorb *et al.*, 1998), carprofen acyl glucuronide (Georges *et al.*, 2000), octanoyl ghrelin (De Vriese, 2007), carbaryl (Sogorb *et al.*, 2004), and nerve agents (Li *et al.*, 2008).

Human plasma contains four esterases: butyrylcholinesterase (BChE) (EC 3.1.1.8), paraoxonase (PON1) (EC 3.1.8.1), acetylcholinesterase (AChE) (EC 3.1.1.7), and albumin esterase (Li *et al.*, 2005). While BChE, AChE, and PON1 are well-known esterases, albumin is not usually included in the esterase family. Albumin does not have an enzyme commission number, which signifies that this protein is considered as lacking a catalytic activity. However, albumin has been conclusively proven to behave as esterase (Erdos and Boggs, 1961; Tove, 1962; Means and Wu, 1979; Hagag *et al.*, 1983; Awad-Elkarim and Means, 1988; Yoshida *et al.*, 1985; Salvi *et al.*, 1997; Sogorb *et al.*, 1998; Watanabe *et al.*, 2000; Kragh-Hansen *et al.*, 2002; Sakurai *et al.*, 2004; Ahmed *et al.*, 2005). Its hydrolytic activity was observed under conditions unfavorable for other blood serum esterases, in particular, in the absence of necessary co-factors (Wilde and Kekwick, 1964), in the presence of specific inhibitors (Casida and Augustinsson, 1959), or after preliminary heating (Córdova *et al.*, 2008). Bobik and colleagues (Bobik *et al.*, 2008) compared the rates for *p*-nitrophenyl acetate hydrolysis in the presence of human serum albumin either expressed in methylotrophic yeast *Pichia pastoris* or isolated from blood. The pseudo-first order rate constant for the hydrolysis of *p*-nitrophenyl acetate in the presence of the recombinant protein ($k_{obs} = (5.5 \pm 0.9) \times 10^{-3}\ s^{-1}$) (Bobik *et al.*, 2008) was similar to that obtained for the blood protein ($k_{obs} = (6.03 \pm 0.7) \times$

10^{-3} s^{-1}) (Watananabe et al., 2000; Matsushita et al., 2004). These results permitted the authors to conclude that the acceleration of ester hydrolysis in the presence of serum albumin is a result of its intrinsic catalytic activity, but not due to the sample contamination with other hydrolases. Despite its hydrolytic activity toward a variety of esters, serum albumin is not considered a genuine hydrolase. First, its turnover numbers (measured by the appearance of the acid product) are too slow for a genuine hydrolase. Second, no proof exists for the presence in serum albumin of the catalytic triad characteristic for hydrolases (Sussman et al., 1993). Therefore, the catalytic activity of serum albumin toward esters tends to be classified as "esterase-like" or "pseudo-esterase" activity.

Although the enzymatic activity of a single molecule of human albumin is low, the concentration of albumin in blood is very high (~0.6 mM), so albumin makes a significant contribution to the drugs pharmacokinetics. For instance, acetylsalicylate (aspirin) hydrolysis is greatly enhanced in the presence of HSA, especially when the drug / HSA mole ratio is low, which confirms the esterase-like activity of HSA (Honma and Ishikawa, 1991). Upon its metabolism in the body, a drug can undergo several types of reactions: hydrolysis, oxidation-reduction, and conjugation with other compounds. Ester bond-containing drugs are usually first hydrolyzed to free OH-group (phase I of drug metabolism), which is then conjugated with endogenous substances, such as glucuronic acid (phase II of drug metabolism). The pattern of acetylsalicylic acid biotransformation is shown in Scheme 2. Although phase I metabolic reactions usually result in decreasing the therapeutic effect of drugs, in some cases, the products of a drug metabolism demonstrate similar or even greater activity (Brown, 2001). For instance, aspirin is characterized by the conversion of the active drug (acetylsalicylic acid) into active metabolite (salicylic acid). Albumin plays a key role in this conversion and thus is regarded as an aspirin esterase (Morikawa et al., 1979). Acetylsalicylic acid was found to acetylate HSA *in vivo* (Burch and Blazer-Yost, 1981; Hawkins et al., 1968; Lighnter et al., 1988; Pinckard et al., 1968) and induce the structural changes in HSA (Hawkins et al., 1969, Yang et al., 2007). Several authors (Walker, 1976, Pinckard et al., 1968; Hawkins et al., 1969) have reported that the protein is acetylated as a result of its interaction with acetylsalicylate under physiologic conditions*in vitro*, and the product formed is stable at pH 10–11. Sequencing of a peptide from HSA, which was radioactively labeled *in vitro* with [1-^{14}C] acetylsalicylic acid, revealed modification of Lys-199 (Walker, 1976). Therefore, Lys-199 has long been considered as the main target of acetyl group transfer, though up to 6 additional radiolabeled peptides were found on the radioautograph of the peptide map of aspirin-treated albumin (Hawkins *et al.*, 1969). The albumin-catalyzed aspirin hydrolysis is believed to occur via the transfer of the acetyl group from aspirin, which is bound to the IIA site of the protein, to the amino group of Lys residue (Scheme 3) (Walker, 1976; Gerig et al., 1981; Yang et al., 2007).

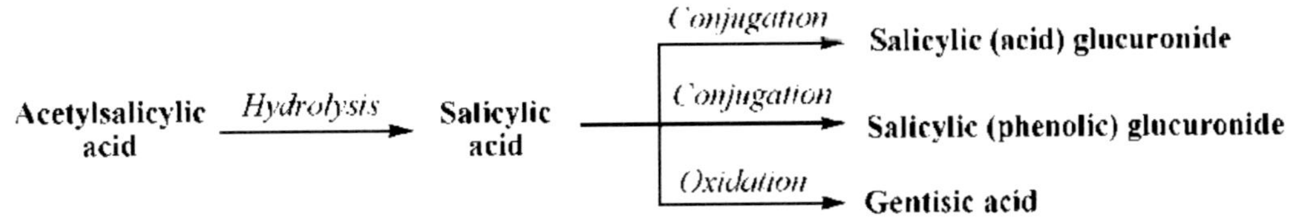

Scheme 2.

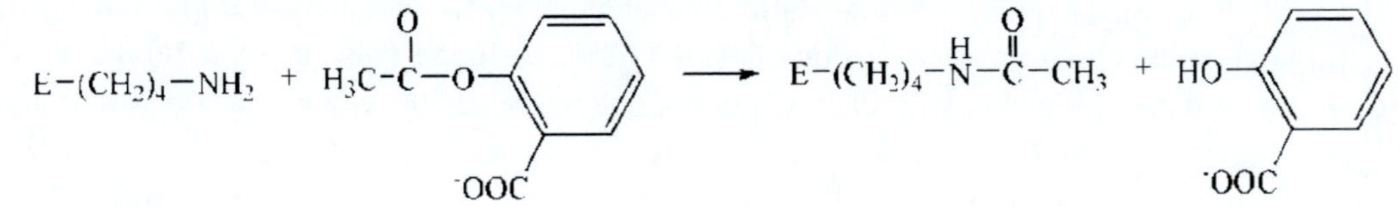

Scheme 3.

It is well-known that Lys-199 is the primary reactive center in HSA. It reacts with different site I ligands via nucleophilic attack on the ligands' carbonyl groups (Walker, 1976; Kurono *et al.*, 1983; Yvon *et al.*, 1988). The ability of Lys-199 to react with acetyl salicylate and penicillins, as well as with arylating agents, is consistent with a pK_a of ~8 for Lys-199 (Gerig and Reinheimer, 1975; Gerig *et al.*, 1978; Kurono *et al.*, 1983; Yvon *et al.*, 1988). The readiness with which Lys-199 can attack certain molecules through nucleophilic substitution is most probably caused by its close location to Lys-195 in the HSA structure (Figure 2).

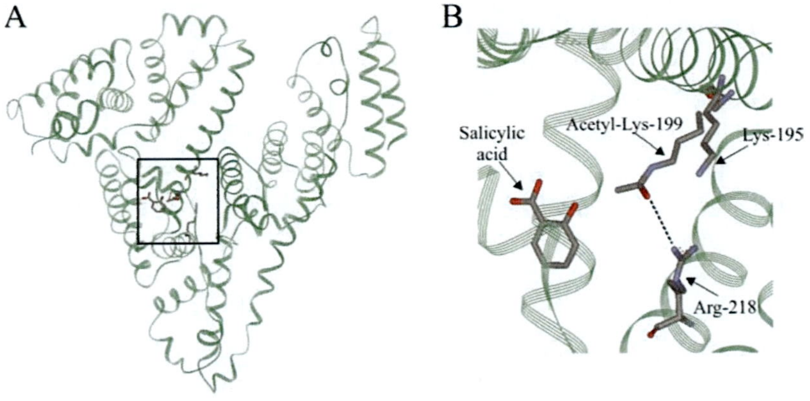

Figure 2.Locations of amino acid residues important for esterase-like activity of HSA toward acetylsalicylic acid. A. The structure of HSA-aspirin complex (Based on the X-ray diffraction structure obtained by Yang et al., 2007, PDB ID 2I2Z). B. The enlarged fragment of HSA shown in a rectangle in panel A. Salycilic acid, acetylated Lys-195, Lys-199 and Arg-218 are shown in stick model.

According to three restrained molecular dynamics simulations of the domain IIA binding site of the HSA, it was concluded that Lys-199 in the basic form is likely connected to the acid form of Lys-195 through a network of H-bonds involving water molecules (Díaz *et al.*, 2001). The presence of these water bridges can be important for stabilizing the configuration of the binding site I and/or promoting a potential Lys-195→Lys-199 proton-transfer process. These results suggest that both Lys-195 and Lys-199, which are situated in subdomain IIA of HSA, could play a combined and comparable chemical role. This model is supported by the fact that the distance between the two residues is relatively short (6.73 Å), as determined by X-ray crystallography (Carter and Ho, 1994; He and Carter, 1992). An unusually low value of pK_a for Lys-199 is also in agreement with the suggested model. Acetylated Lys-199 is close to Arg-218, Trp-214, Leu-238, and His-242 in the pocket (Yang *et al.*, 2007). The acetyl group of acetyl lysine is surrounded by Trp-214 and Arg-218 and forms a hydrogen bond with Arg-218 (3.26 Å) (Figure 2B). Compared with the position of Lys-199 in HSA-myristate, the side chain of acetylated Lys-199 in HSA-myristate-aspirin complex stretches out to place the amino group of Lys-199 toward the hydroxyl group of salicylic acid.

Although there are some conformational changes of the side chains located in the aspirin-binding site, the acetylation of Lys-199 of HSA does not cause overall changes in the secondary structures of HSA (Yang *et al.*, 2007). Salicylate interacts with the same site of the protein's globule as the initial substrate, but its conformation in the crystalline structure of HSA-aspirin differs from that in an HSA-salicylic acid complex. Besides, salicylic acid forms more contacts with functional groups of albumin's active center than its acetylated derivative. This fact may explain the enhanced affinity of HSA to salicylate as compared to acetylsalicylate (Honma and Ishikawa, 1991) and inhibitory action of salicylic acid on the albumin-catalyzed hydrolysis of aspirin.

Recently, studies with acetylsalicylic acidas a substrate have showed that, although Lys-199 is important, other lysine residues become acetylated as a result of the aspirin pseudo-esterase activity of human albumin (Liyasova *et al.*, 2010). The analysis of tryptic peptides obtained from HSA, which was acetylated with 0.3 mM aspirin for 24 h, by LC/MS/MS and MALDI-TOF/TOF mass spectrometry revealed four modified lysines: Lys-199, Lys-402, Lys-519, and Lys-545. High concentrations of aspirin (20 mM) resulted in acetylation of 26 albumin's lysine residues. However, this high degree of acetylation is not likely to occur *in vivo*, since a 20 mM aspirin concentration is well beyond the therapeutic blood level. In addition, the metabolite of aspirin, salicylic acid, in concentration greater than 5.4 mM causes severetoxicity (Dargan *et al.*, 2002).

Acetylated lysine is stable for at least 21 days at pH 7.4, 37 °C (Liyasova *et al.*, 2010). Assuming that albumin's half-life in the blood is about 20 days (Peters, Jr. T., 1996), it can be anticipated that once it becomes acetylated, albumin remains acetylated for the rest of its life-time in the circulation. This idea is supported by the striking finding of a small amount of acetylated albumin in a commercial albumin preparation, which indicates that albumin does not lose the acetyl group even under the conditions of industrial isolation (Liyasova *et al.*, 2010).

The biological consequences of albumin's acetylation *in vivo* are not fully understood. Considering the widespread use of aspirin by children and adults, investigation into the consequences of the acetylation of albumin on various functions of albumin *in vivo* is of interest. Previous findings suggested that this phenomenon may be of significance (Minden and Farr, 1967). There is increasing evidence that aspirin differs significantly from other salicylates in its effects on homeostasis in human (Quike, 1966a; Quike, 1966b). The acetyl group of aspirin appears to be implicated in many physiologic phenomena (Brown, 2001). The syndrome of aspirin resistance characterized by asthma, rhinitis, and nasal polyps (Samter and Beers, 1967) is induced by aspirin but not other salicylates. The unique ability of aspirin to form acetyl derivatives of human proteins and other body constituents may play a role in these reactions. Binding of aspirin to human albumin was shown to reduce prostaglandins binding to albumin (Attallah and Lee, 1980). In addition, acetylation of albumin by aspirin was demonstrated to inhibit bilirubin binding (Trynda *et al.*, 1990). Therefore, modification of HSA by aspirin may alter albumin's traditional roles in binding endogenous and exogenous compounds and eventually affect drugs pharmacokinetics.

It was concluded that the aspirin esterase activity of albumin is a pseudo-esterase activity, since salicylate is formed due to the reaction of acetylsalicylic acid with the protein's lysine residues yielding stably acetylates lysines. In this reaction, albumin is more like a reagent than a catalyst, since its reactive sites cannot be easily regenerated for the next round of reactions. Indeed, albumin acetylated by aspirin has the reduced esterase activity with β-naphtyl acetate, as demonstrated in the experiments on in-gel esterase activity (Liyasova *et al.*, 2010).

Interestingly, Tyr-411 was found not to play a role in the reaction between human albumin and aspirin, while this site was shown to be important in the hydrolysis of other acetyl-containing agents (Watanabe *et al.*, 2000; Sakurai, *et al.*, 2004; Lockridge *et al.*, 2008). Indeed, the protein's subdomain IIIA containing Tyr-411 has been linked to a well-known esterase-like activity toward such substrates as *p*-nitrophenyl acetate (Watanabe *et al.*, 2000) and several *N*-carbobenzoxy-D(L)-alanine *p*-nitrophenyl esters (Kurono *et al.*, 1992). Site-directed mutagenesis studies have shown that Arg-410 and Tyr-411 are essential for the esterase-like activity of HSA toward *p*-nitrophenyl acetate, and the reaction mechanism similar to that of proteases has been suggested (Watanabe *et al.*, 2000; Sakurai, *et al.*, 2004).

The hydrolytic activity toward *p*-nitrophenyl acetate has been studied in detail using several rHSA mutants including one containing Ser-411. The obtained results indicate that the presence of a hydroxyl group in position 411 and the nature of its immediate surroundings are crucial for the esterase-like activity of HSA (Watanabe *et al.*, 2000). For instance, substitution of Arg-410 with alanine resulted in the decrease of the catalytic activity to 12 % of that for native protein. A minor activity (~21 % of activity) could be registered when serine, but not alanine or phenylalanine, was present at position 411 (Watanabe *et al.*, 2000).

The esterase-like activity of HSA toward *p*-nitrophenyl acetate was mainly linked to the protein's domain IIIA, where Tyr-411 is situated. To determine the location of albumin's active sites and clarify the mechanisms underlying its ligand-binding and enzyme-like properties, Matsushita and colleagueshave used *Pichia pastoris* to separately express the three recombinant domains of HSA (Matsushita *et al*, 2004). The catalytic activity of rHSA and individual domains with respect to *p*-nitrophenyl acetate is shown in Table 2.

Table 2. Hydrolysis rate constants (k_{obs}) for *p*-nitrophenyl acetate*

HSA or its individual domains	K_{obs} (s × 10^{-3})
rHSA	7.13 ± 0.90
Domain I	1.73 ± 0.65
Domain II	ND
Domain III	3.18 ± 0.83

*The reaction mixture contained 5 μM *p*-nitrophenyl acetate and 20 μM rHSA or individual domains in 67 mM phosphate buffer (ph 7.4 and 25 ^{0}C). All values are mean± SD (n = 5 to 7).ND, not detectable (Matsushita *et al*, 2004).

The highest esterase-like activity was detected in domain III, where site II is located, but this activity was about 45% of that of rHSA. Some activity was also detected in domain I, although it was much weaker than that of domain III (Table 2). This suggests that interdomain interaction is crucial for the full esterase-like activity of HSA. No enzymatic activity was detected for domain II, suggesting the absence of an active site in this domain. This finding is consistent with the fact that domain II has not been reported to possess esterase-like activity in studies of intact HSA. The esterase-like activity of HSA in subdomain IIIA is due to the close proximity of Arg-410 and Tyr-411 (Figure 3). In the crystal structure of the protein, the distance between the reactive group of the tyrosine residue and the nitrogen atoms of the arginine residue is only 2-3 Å (He and Carter, 1992; Ahmed *et al.*, 2005). When HSA was minimally modified with methylglyoxal, tryptic peptide mapping indicated a hotspot of modification at Arg-410 located in drug-binding site II and the active site of albumin-associated esterase activity (Ahmed *et al.*, 2005).

Similar to the reaction with aspirin, HSA-catalyzed hydrolysis of *p*-nitrophenyl acetate was shown to proceed via covalent acyl-protein intermediate. First, it was demonstrated by the formation of radioactively labeled HSA upon its reaction with [^{14}C]-labeled nitrophenyl acetate (Means and Bender, 1975). Radioactivity was firmly bound to the protein and could not be removed by extensive dialysis. Later (Lockridge *et al.*, 2008), MALDI-TOF mass spectrometry data revealed that Tyr-411 was modified in the reaction.

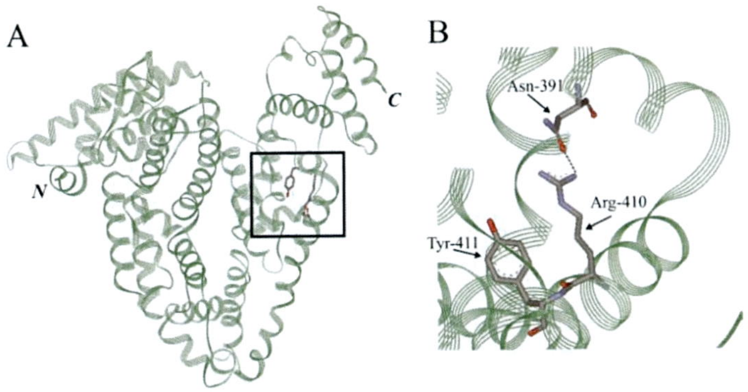

Figure 3.The location of amino acid residues important for esterase-like activity of HSA toward *p*-nitrophenyl acetate. A. The structure of HSA (Based on the X-ray diffraction structure obtained by Sugio *et al.*, 1999, PDB ID 1AO6). B. The enlarged fragment of HSA shown in a rectangle in panel A. Asn-391, Arg-410 and Tyr-411 are shown in stick model.

Transfer of a substrate's acyl residue to serum albumin in the course of the protein-catalyzed ester hydrolysis is similar to the event that occurs in the course of nucleophilic catalysis of peptide- and ester-bonds hydrolysis by serine proteases. At the same time, several essential differences have been revealed, which demonstrate the imperfectness of albumin as a catalyst in comparison with real enzymes. In particular, general acid-base catalysis plays an essential role in serine proteases providing the activation of a hydroxyl group of serine, which is usually inert under physiological conditions, for nucleophilic attack on a substrate and subsequent water molecule activation (Scheme 4) (Branden and Tooze, 1991).

The key element of the catalysis by the enzyme is the proton transfer from the serine's hydroxyl group to the nitrogen atom of the histidine's imidazole ring. This provides the negative charge at the oxygen atom of serine, which favors its attack on the substrate's carbon leading to the formation of a tetrahedral intermediate (1). The positive charge in the so-called "oxyanion hole" in the enzyme's active center plays an essential role for the intermediate's stabilization. Thc next step is the proton transfer from histidine to the oxygen of the leaving group, removal of the reaction product (alcohol R_1OH) and the formation of acyl-enzyme intermediate. Now histidine residue becomes capable of serving as a general base and withdrawing a proton from the water molecule, which occupies the site of the removed alcohol in the enzyme's active center. The formed anion OH^- undergoes nucleophilic attack on the carbonylic carbon atom of acyl-enzyme, thus forming a new intermediate (3). The following proton transfer to the serine's oxygen results in the release of acyl product and regeneration of serine residue for a subsequent catalytic round.

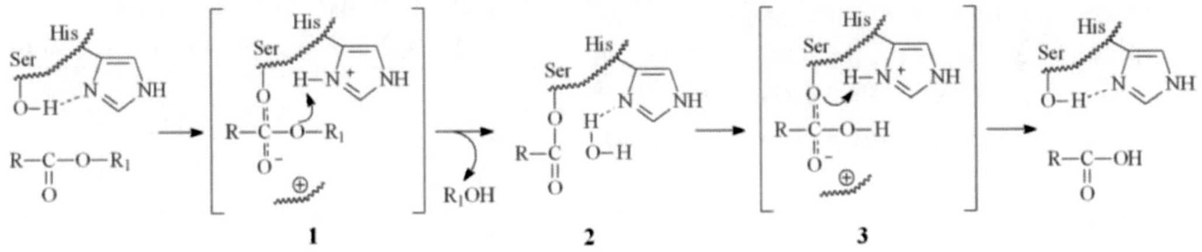

Scheme 4.

Albumin catalyzes the same reaction without participation of a proton transfer system that is typical for serine proteases. This statement is supported by the absence of the deuterium isotopic effect for ester hydrolysis in the presence of HSA (Lockridge *et al.*, 2008). Authors (Ahmed *et al.*, 2005) studied the pH dependence of esterase activity of HSA. The obtained pH profile demonstrated that an amino acid residue involved in the catalysis has a pK_a of 7.9 ± 0.1. This is assigned to the ionization of the Tyr-411 phenolic group, lowered by the positive electrostatic interaction with Arg-410. Crystallographic and mutational studies have indicated that Arg-410 is located in drug-binding site II of HSA, which is situated in subdomain IIIA (Watanabe *et al.*, 2000; Petitpas *et al.*, 2001). In the native state, the guanidine nitrogen of Arg-410 is hydrogen-bonded to the side chain carbonyl group of Asn-391 (bond length is1.9 Å) (Scheme 5, Figure 3). Molecular simulations with the phenoxide anion of Tyr-411 indicated electrostatic interaction of the Arg-410 guanidinium and Tyr-411 phenoxide groups: with energy minimization, the distance between Arg-410 guanidinium ω-NH and Tyr-410 phenoxide –O$^-$ is predicted to be 2.0 Å (Ahmed *et al.*, 2005). To model the transition state structure of the esterase reaction, authors positioned the carbonyl carbon of the synthetic substrate, *p*-nitrophenyl acetate, close to the phenoxide catalytic base of Tyr-411 (bond length is1.44 Å). Energy minimized molecular dynamics studies predicted hydrogen bonding between the guanidine hydrogen of Arg-410 and carbonyl oxygen in the substrate (bond length is2.3 Å). Electrostatic interaction also stabilizes the increasing negative charge on the substrate's carbonyl oxygen during the nucleophilic attack of Tyr-411 (Scheme 5). In the putative acyl-protein intermediate with *O*-acetylated Tyr-411, the acetyl carbonyl oxygen forms a hydrogen bond with the guanidine group of Arg-410 (bond length is ~2.3 Å). At the same time, Arg-410 remains hydrogen-bonded to Asn-391 throughout the catalytic reaction. This supports the suggestion that a catalytic triad of amino acid residues Tyr-411, Arg-410, and Asn-391 sustains esterase activity of HSA (Scheme 5) (Ahmed *et al.*, 2005).

It is noteworthy that the efficiency of *p*-nitrophenyl acetate hydrolysis is inversely proportional to the basicity of the reactive amino acid residue of albumin from different sources. The pK_a value of Tyr-411 of HSA is unusually low (8.7, according to Means and Bender, 1975, or 9.2, according to Sakurai *et al.*, 2004). The correspondent values for catalytically active tyrosine residues of bovine, rabbit, rat and equine serum albumins are 9.3, 9.4, 9.5 and 9.7, respectively (Sakurai *et al.*, 2004). Since the increase of ionization constant for OH group corresponds to the decrease in the relative amount of the highly nucleophilic deprotonated form of the amino acid, it may be concluded that the hydrolytic activity of albumin depends both on the basicity and nucleophilicity of the protein's tyrosine residue. Since the proton transfer system that is able to activate the water molecule is absent in the albumin's reaction center, deacylation of the covalent acyl-protein adduct (2) proceeds most probably via nucleophilic attack of the hydroxyl ion (Scheme 6).

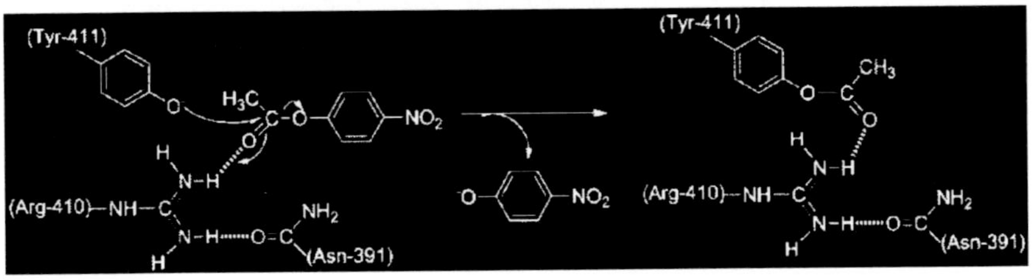

Scheme 5.

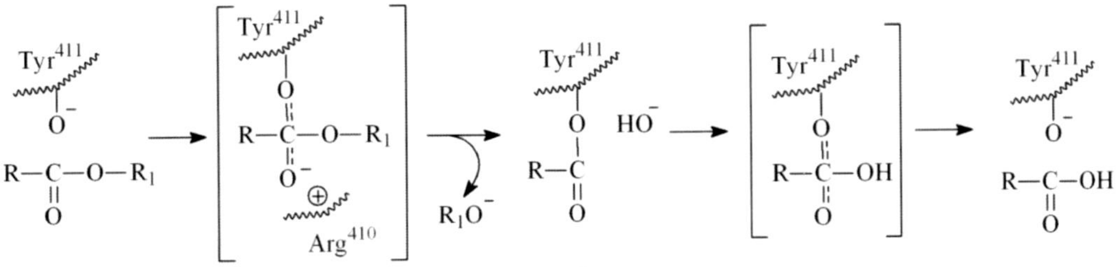

1 2

Scheme 6.

Why does aspirin behave differently from other phenyl esters? The authors (Liyasova *et al.*, 2010) provided an explanation for the well-known fact. According to the model suggested by Sakurai (Sakurai *et al.*, 2004), the side chain of Arg-410 forms a hydrogen bond with the carbonyl oxygen of the ester, thus facilitating nucleophilic attack by the phenolic oxygen of Tyr-411 on the carbonyl carbon of the ester. However, in the case of aspirin, the reaction may be complicated by the presence of a carboxylic group. Therefore, it is possible that the carboxylic oxygens rather than the carbonyl oxygen of the acetyl group interact with Arg-410, making the acetylation of Tyr-411 impossible due to a wrong orientation of the aspirin molecule.

Human albumin is believed to hydrolyze esters because multiple equivalents of product are formed for each equivalent of albumin. The above comparison demonstrates that serum albumin, though able to catalyze ester hydrolysis, is a less favorable biological catalyst under physiological conditions than natural hydrolases. Esterase-like activity of albumin toward *p*-nitrophenyl acetate has been attributed to the turnover at tyrosine 411. The half-life for deacetylation of Tyr-411 at pH 8.0, 22 °C was 61 ± 4 h. This very slow deacetylation rate (k = 0.0002 min^{-1}) confirms a previous report that deacetylation is the rate-limiting step for the reaction of human albumin with *p*-nitrophenyl acetate (Masson *et al.*, 2007). Since hydroxyl anion is necessary for the regeneration of the reactive tyrosine residue, acyl-albumin adduct is highly stable under conditions near physioliogical (Lockridge *et al.*, 2008).

Recent studies with *p*-nitrophenyl acetate as a substrate have showed that, although Tyr-411 is important, the pseudo-esterase activity of human albumin is also dependent on the presence of different amino acid residues (Lockridge *et al.*, 2008).*p*-Nitrophenyl acetate creates multiple stable acetylated adducts, a property contrary to the turnover. The degree of the protein's acetylation depends on the concentration of *p*-nitrophenyl acetate and the time of incubation. Only Tyr-411 was acetylated within the first 5 min of reaction with 0.5 mM *p*-nitrophenyl acetate. Prolonged incubation (0.5-6 h) resulted in the partial acetylation of 16-17 residues including Asp-1, Lys-4, Lys-12, Tyr-411, Lys-413, and Lys-414 (Figure 4A). Higher concentration of *p*-nitrophenyl acetate (10 mM) gave rise to the acetylation of 59 lysines, 10 serines, 8 threonines, 4 tyrosines, and Asp-1 (Figure 4B). This finding allowed the authors to suggest that the majority of the "esterase" activity of albumin is due to the reaction of the substrate with lysines, serines, threonines and tyrosines of the protein. These acetylated residues do not turnover but form stable adducts. Therefore, after 82 residues had been acetylated, esterase activity is almost completely inhibited (Lockridge *et al.*, 2008).

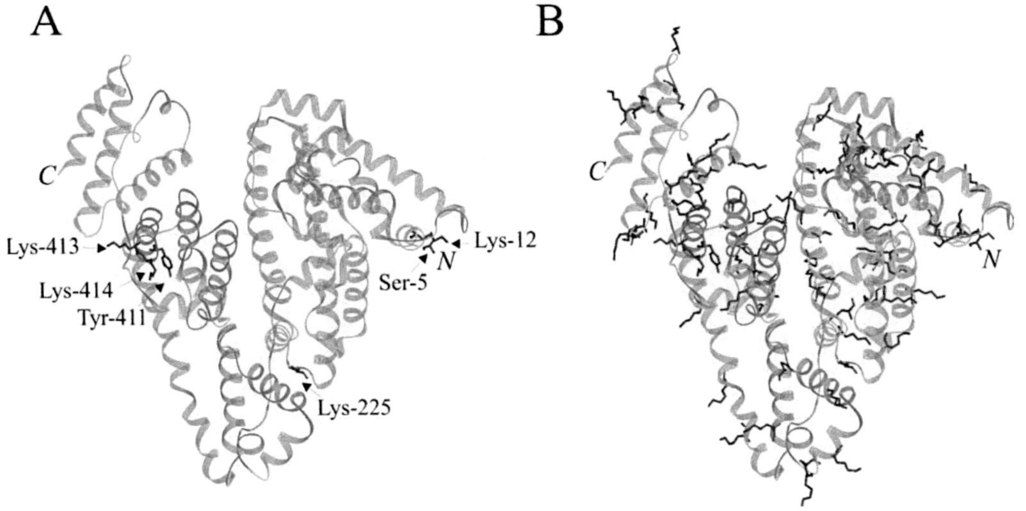

Figure 4.Location of amino acid residues in human albumin, which were acetylated upon the protein's interaction with *p*-nitrophenyl acetate (Lockridge *et al.*, 2008). Asp-1 and Lys-4 are missing from the structure. Based on the X-ray diffraction structure obtained by Sugio *et al.*, 1999, PDB ID 1AO6. A. Incubation of HSA (15 μM) with 0.5 mM *p*-nitrophenyl acetate. B. Incubation of HSA (15 μM) with 10 mM *p*-nitrophenyl acetate.

Additional support for the conclusion that lysines and tyrosine participate in the pseudo-esterase activity of albumin comes from studies of albumin modified by acyl glucuronides (Qiu *et al.*, 1998; Williams and Dickinson, 1994; Zia-Amirhosseini *et al.*, 1995; Dubois-Presle *et al.*, 1994; Dubois-Presle *et al.*, 1996; Georges *et al.*, 1999; Georges *et al.*, 2000; Greige-Georges *et al.*, 2003). The formation of acyl glucuronides, which are then excreted into urine, is a major metabolic pathway for many compounds with a carboxylic acid function. Metabolites of this kind are reactive electrophilic species and thus not only reversible bind to HSA, but also covalently react with the protein both *in vitro* and *in vivo*. For example, as a result of albumin incubation with acylglucuronides of non-steroidal anti-inflammatory drugs of the series of phenylpropionates, three types of albumin adducts were observed (Georges *et al.*, 1999). Two mechanisms have been proposed for these covalent interactions (Qiu *et al.*, 1998; Williams and Dickinson, 1994; Zia-Amirhosseini *et al.*, 1995). One is a displacement mechanism in which a nucleophilic group (NH_2 or -OH) of the protein attacks the acyl carbon of the aglycone, displacing the glucuronic acid and forming an amide or ester bond between the protein and the drug (a transacylation mechanism). The other involves the migration of the acyl group from the position 1 to the position 2, 3, or 4 of the sugar, ring-chain tautomerism of the pyranose ring, and, finally, condensation of the aldehyde group of the ring-opened tautomer with a lysine ε-amino group on the protein to form an imine (a glycation mechanism). Subsequent Amadori rearrangement of the imine can give a more stable ketoamine derivative. Thus, in the latter mechanism, glucuronic acid is not displaced but instead acts as a bridge between the protein and the drug moiety. Presumably, one or both of these mechanisms may be involved in the formation of protein adducts *in vivo*.

The reactivity of *R*- and *S*-carprofen acylglucuronides (Figure 5) toward HSA was investigated *in vitro* (Georges *et al.*, 2000; Greige-Georges *et al.*, 2003). The irreversible binding of these metabolites to the HSA occurred at physiological pH and 37 °Cinstantaneously and stereoselectively in favor of the *R*-enantiomer glucuroide. The amount of carprofen adducts remained stable with time up to 48 h and increased with the glucuronide concentration. The addition of imine-trapping reagents did not affect the modification, which supports the suggestion that the reaction is not mediated by a Schiff base mechanism. Moreover, the extreme rapidity of the covalent binding supports a mechanism of nucleophilic attack. Competition studies with ligands specific to different HSA sites indicated that carprofen glucuronides interacted mainly with site II. The modification of HSA by amino acid-specific chemicals led to the conclusion that Tyr, Lys or Arg residues in site II were mainly involved (Greige-Georges *et al.*, 2003).

The hydrolysis of the conjugates of both enantiomers was accelerated in the presence of HSA (Georges *et al.*, 2000). However, the increase in the rate of hydrolysis of *S*-carprofen glucuronide was more profound, so the hydrolysis was stereoselective in favor of the *S*-enantiomer. *R*-carprofen glucuronide was protected by the protein from migration, which increased its overall stability (Georges *et al.*, 2000). The protein domains and the amino acid residues likely to be responsible for the hydrolytic activity of HSA were deduced from the results of various investigations. Dansylsarcosine, a specific ligand of the domain II of HSA, impaired the hydrolysis, whereas dansylamide and digoxin, which are specific ligands of domaines I and III, respectively, had no effect. The extent of the binding of *R*-carprofen glucuronide and the rate of its hydrolysis by HSA increased with pH, indicating the participation of basic amino acids in this process. The results obtained with chemically modified HSA suggest that Tyr and Lys residues of the protein are mainly involved in the hydrolysis of *S*-carprofen glucuronide, while Lys residues are important for the hydrolysis of its diastereoisomer.

HSA enantioselectivity is clearly demonstrated by the tendency of the protein to preferentially recognize one of ester enantiomers. The stereoselectivity of albumin toward the hydrolysis of acylglucuronides depends on the aglycone's nature. In contrast to carprofen glucuronide isomers (Georges *et al.*, 2000; Greige-Georges *et al.*, 2003), the *R*-ketoprofen glucuronide (Figure 5) was a better substrate for albumin's catalytic activity than its *S*-stereomer (Dubois-Presle *et al.*, 1995). It was apparent (Hayball *et al.*, 1992) that albumin, rather than plasma esterases, catalyzed the hydrolysis of ketoprofen glucuronides *in vivo*. The mean hydrolysis half-life of *R*-ketoprofen glucuronide in plasma at physiological pH and temperature was 1.37 ± 0.30 h. The corresponding value for *S*-ketoprofen glucuronide, 3.46 ± 0.84 hr, was significantly different ($P < 0.005$). *S*-Ketoprofen glucuronide was more avidly bound to the protein at the physiological concentration of HSA. However, in more dilute HSA solutions, the preferential binding of *S*-isomer was not so obvious. Based on the data on the binding and hydrolysis of ketoprofen glucuronides by HSA, the authors (Hayball *et al.*, 1992) proposed the existence of separate binding and catalytic sites on the albumin molecule for these metabolites.

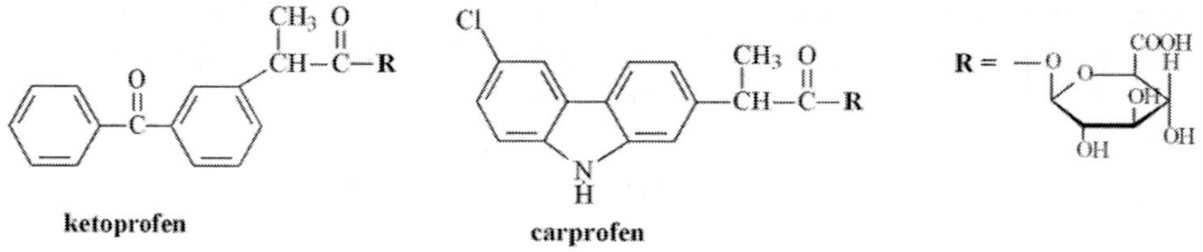

Figure 5.Structure of acylglucoronides of non-steroidal anti-inflammatory drugs interacting with HSA.

A number of acidic non-steroidal anti-inflammatory drugs have elicited potentially fatal hypersensitivity reactions (including anaphylaxis, bronchospasm and hepatotoxicity). The authors (Zia-Amirhosseine *et al.*, 1995) hypothesized that the allergic-like reactions and the organ toxicities may occur via an immune-based mechanism whereby the acyl glucuronide metabolites of drugs act as haptens upon covalent binding to a serum albumin.

From the pharmaceutical and clinical points of view, it is interesting that the esterase-like activity of HSA can be used to activate pro-drugs. For example, a novel angiotensin II receptor antagonist olmesartan medoxomil [CS-866: (5-methyl-2-oxo-1,3-dioxolen-4-yl) methoxy-4-(1-hydroxyl)-2-propyl-1-{4-[2-(tetrazol-5-yl)-phenyl]phenyl}methylimidazol-5-carboxylate] is activated in human plasma with a half-life of a few seconds. The activation occurs through its hydrolysis to the active drug olmesartan (RNH-6270) (Ikeda, 2000; Koike *et al.*, 2001; Brousil and Burke, 2003; Ma *et al.*, 2005) (Scheme 7). The serum from other organisms can also activate the pro-drug. Among the five species studied (Ikeda, 2000), the hydrolytic activity towards CS-866 was the highest in rabbit serum and decreased in the following order: dogs>mice>rats>humans.Serum albumin plays a key role in the activation of olmesartan medoxomil. *Ma* and coworkers (Ma *et al.*, 2005) have shown that HSA is able to hydrolyze the pro-drug *in vitro*. Warfarin (site I drug) and ibuprofen (site II drug) acted as competitive inhibitors of hydrolysis of the pro-drug, whereas *n*-butyl-*p*-aminobenzoate, and diazepam did not. All of the mutant HSAs tested (K199A, W214A, and Y411A) exhibited a significant decrease in reactivity, suggesting that Lys-199, Trp-214, and Tyr-411 play important roles in the hydrolysis. These findings suggest that HSA has two catalytic sites for CS-866.

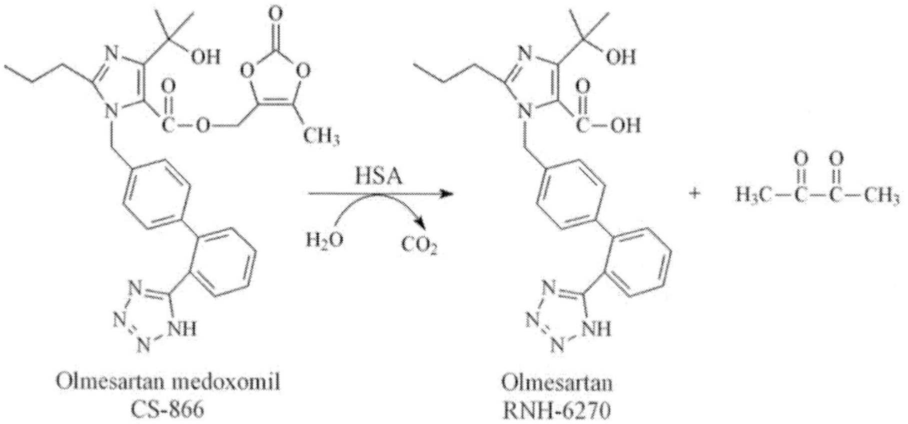

Scheme 7.

The possibility of CS-866 binding in sites I and II is supported by computer modeling data for the interaction of albumin with the drug molecule (Ma *et al.*, 2005). In site I, the carbonyl oxygen atom of the ester moiety forms a hydrogen bond with the side chain of Lys-199, and this hydrogen bond can function as an oxyanion hole. The importance of Lys-199 indicated by the model is consistent with the decreased hydrolytic activity of the K199A mutant and the HSA variant produced by chemical modification of Lys. The catalytic residue may be Glu-292; the distance between the oxygen atom of the side chain of Glu-292 and the carbonyl carbon of the ester moiety of CS-866 is 4.8 Å. The hydrophobic interaction between CS-866 and Trp-214 indicated by the model is consistent with the diminished hydrolytic activity of the W214A mutant and the HSA variant produced by chemical modification of Trp.

In accordance with the second model, CS-866 was placed in site II using the pocket for myristate-4 (Curry *et al.*, 1998). The distance between the hydroxyl oxygen atom of Tyr-411 and the carbonyl carbon of the moiety of CS-866 is 3.3 Å, which suggests the possibility that Tyr-411 serves as a catalytic residue. The importance of Tyr-411 and Lys-414 is consistent with the decreased hydrolytic activity of the Y411A mutant and of the HSA variants produced by chemical modification of Tyr or Lys. Model II indicates that the mechanism of hydrolysis of CS-866 is almost the same as that found in previous studies for *p*-nitrophenyl esters, with the exception of the involvement of Arg-410 (Watanabe *et al.*, 2000; Sakurai *et al.*, 2004).

The hydrolysis of CS-866 by HSA followed Michaelis-Menten kinetics. Compared with the release of *p*-nitrophenol from *p*-nitrophenyl acetate, CS-866 showed lower affinity to HSA and a lower catalytic rate of hydrolysis (Table 3). That is, compared to CS-866, *p*-nitrophenyl acetate has a structure and orientation that are better suited for the hydrolysis by HSA. Detoxification of organophosphates, carbamates and pyrethroids in the body occurs mainly through their hydrolysis (Sogorb and Vilanova, 2002). The esterases involved in the hydrolysis of these compounds have been intensively studied, and their biochemical and toxicological characterizations in mammals have been performed. The two main enzyme groups involved in the hydrolysis of these toxicants are phosphotriesterases (PTEs) and carboxylesterases (CbEs) (Sogorb and Vilanova, 2002). Serum albumins are also known to bind organophosphates and carbamates (Mourik and de Jong, 1978; Maliwal and Guthrie, 1981; Silva *et al.*, 2004) and react with them (Sanger, 1963; Means and Wu, 1979; Black *et al.*, 1999). Some phosphoroorganic compounds that interact with serum albumin are depicted in Figure 6. Using equilibrium dialysis, Mourik and Jong (Mourik and de Jong, 1978) showed that binding constants for the interaction of HSA or BSA with ethyl parathion at pH 7.2 and 4 °C were of the order of 10^6 M^{-1}. For paraoxon, the parathion oxygen analogue, these constants were considerably lower, in the order of magnitude of 10^3 M^{-1} for BSA and 10^4 M^{-1} for HSA. The authors concluded that the great difference in affinity of serum albumin to parathion and its metabolite paraoxon is, in part, responsible for high toxicity of parathion, since conversion of parathion into paraoxon in the liver not only leads to a more potent inhibitor of cholinesterases, but also increases the level of free organophosphate in plasma.

Using the same method, other authors (Sultatos *at el.*, 1984) have found that fatty acids-free BSA binds parathion and chlorpyrifos with $K_a = (9.0 \pm 0.2) \times 10^4$ M^{-1} and $K_a = (29.4 \pm 0.8) \times 10^4$ M^1, respectively. The studied substances are reversibly bound in the same site. Only one insecticide molecule can be bound per protein molecule. Interaction of serum albumins with oxygen analoges of such insecticides as chlorpyrifos and paraoxon results in the hydrolysis of a phosphodiester bond in these compounds (Scheme 8) (Sultatos *at el.*, 1984; Ortigoza-Ferado *et al.*, 1984).

Table 3.Kinetic parameters for the hydrolysis of CS-866 and *p*-nitrophenyl acetate by HSAat pH 7.4 and 25 °C

Substrate	k_{cat},10^{-3} s^{-1}	K_s,μM	k_{cat}/K_s,M^{-1} s^{-1}
CS-866[a]	0.845	42.5	19.9
p-nitrophenyl acetate[b]	86.8	217	403.4

[a]data from Ma et al., 2005
[b]data from Sakura et al., 2004

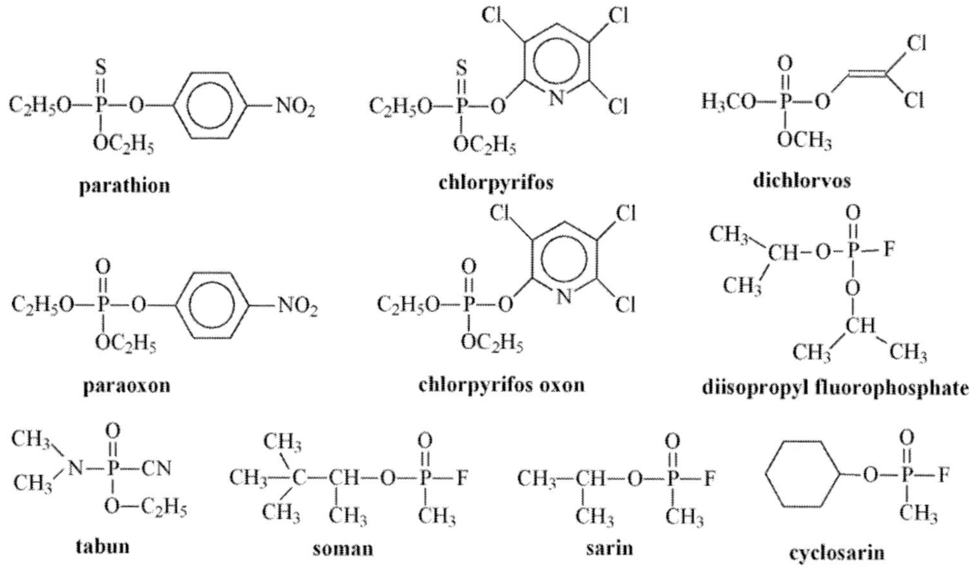

Figure 6.Structures of some phosphoroorganic compounds that interact with serum albumin.

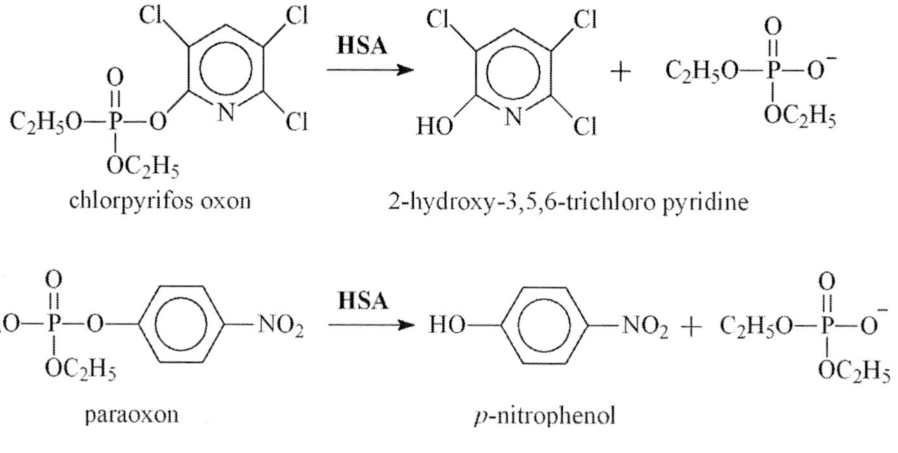

Scheme 8.

The suggestion that albumin itself (or a factor closely associated with albumin) actually hydrolyzes paraoxone was first proposed by Erdos and Boggs, who reported two paraoxonase activities present in human serum (Erdos and Boggs, 1961). In many studies on the enzymatic activities associated with albumin, it was not clear if the activities were associated with the albumin molecule itself, or were associated with minor proteins that co-fractionated with albumin (Taylor, 1977). It was observed that the albumin-associated paraoxonase activity was partially inhibited by NaCl and was not present in serum obtained from an analbuminemic individual (Ortigoza-Ferado *et al.*, 1984). This data suggested that albumin itself, rather than a protein bound to or co-fractionated with albumin, mediates paraoxonase activity. Esterase-like activity of albumin to phosphoroorganic compounds, unlike other known phosphotriesterases, is not sensitive to EDTA (Sultatos *at el.*, 1984; Ortigoza-Ferado *et al.*, 1984).

It was shown that there is a phosphotriesterase in chiken serum (Diaz-Alejo *et al.*, 1998; Sogorb *et al.*, 1993; Sogorb *et al.*, 1998). This phosphotriesterase was able to hydrolyse *O*-alkyl *O*-2,5-dichlorophenyl phosphoramidates in a non-stereospecific way (Diaz-Alejo *et al.*, 1998). The phosphotriesterase activity was not Ca^{2+}-dependent (Sogorb *et al.*, 1993) and was not inhibited by EDTA (Sogorb *et al.*, 1993). This activity was activated by Cu^{2+} (Sogorb *et al.*, 1993). After purification to homogeneity, the phosphotriesterase activity was found to be associated with albumin (Sogorb *et al.*, 1998). Chicken serum albumin (CSA) also hydrolyzed*p*-nitrophenyl butyrate, but was unable to hydrolyze paraoxon (Sogorb *et al.*, 1998). Studies by Sogorb *et al.* (Sogorb *et al.*, 1998; Sogorb *et al.*, 1999) reported phosphotriesterase activity associated with human, chicken, rabbit, bovine serum albumin and recombinant human serum albumin. The hydrolysis of several *O*-alkyl *O*-2,5-dichlorophenyl phosphoramidates by these proteins was observed. The authors have proposed that such proteins should be termed AB-esterases, since it is likely that the hydrolysis proceeds through a covalent phosphylated intermediate, which then undergoes dephosphylation, exhibiting intermediate behavior between the A- and B-type esterases. According Aldridge classification (Aldridge, 1953), A-esterases hydrolyze carboxyl esters and organophosphorus compounds without being inhibited by the latter. B-esterases likewise hydrolyze carboxyl esters and organophosphorus compounds, but are inhibited by the latter. In the case of the type B carboxyl esterases, the organophosphorus compounds act as suicide substrates, and the interaction between carboxyl esterase and organophosphorus compound results in the irreversible inhibition by phosphorylation of a serine group within the active site of the enzyme (Aldridge and Reiner, 1972). B-esterases may also be regarded as proteins involved in organophosphorus compounds detoxification because each molecule of a B-esterase is able to react with an organophosphorus molecule, scavenging the latter and thus preventing it from reaching its targets within the central nervous system.

Organophosphates and carbamates are actually hydrolyzed by albumin through transient phosphylation/alkylation of its active site (De Bisschop *et al.*, 1987; Sogorb *et al.*, 1998; Sogorb and Vilanova, 2002; Sogorb *et al.*, 2004; Sogorb *et al.*, 2007). Tyr-411 of human serum albumin is an established site for the covalent attachment of 10-fluoroethoxyphosphonyl-*N*-biotinamidopentyldecanamide, diisopropylfluorophosphate, chlorpyrifos oxon, soman, sarin, and dichlorvos (Sanger, 1963; Means and Wu, 1979; Black *et al.*, 1999; Sogorb *et al.*, 2004; Adams *et al.*, 2004; Schopfer *et al.*, 2005; Li *et al.*, 2007; Li *et al.*, 2008). Albumin was shown to covalently bind radiolabeled diisopropylfluorophosphate (DFP) (Means and Wu, 1979). $DF^{32}P$-labeling of human albumin followed by peptide sequencing showed that the labeled tyrosine is in the tetrapeptide sequence Arg-*Tyr*-Thr-Lys (Sanger, 1963). Later, when the complete amino acid sequence of human albumin was known, the active site tyrosine was identified as Tyr-411. Arg and Tyr were subsequently identified as Arg-410 and Tyr-411, the key residues of the esterase–like activity of HSA (Watanabe *et al.*, 2000). Mass spectrometry (MS) identified Tyr-410 of bovine albumin (equivalent to Tyr-411 of human albumin) as the covalent binding site for fluorophosphinate linked to biotin via a 17-atom spacer (FP-biotin, Figure 7) (Schopfer *et al.*, 2005). *In vitro* pre-treatment of plasma with a variety of organophosphates (chlorpyrifos oxon, echothiophate, malaoxon, paraoxon, methyl paraoxon, diazoxon, diisopropylfluorophosphate, and dichlorvos) reduced the subsequent reaction of FP-biotin with albumin, indicating that all of these organophosphates also react with albumin (Peeples *et al.*, 2005). These observations strongly suggest that albumin is also a scavenger for these organophosphates *in vivo*.

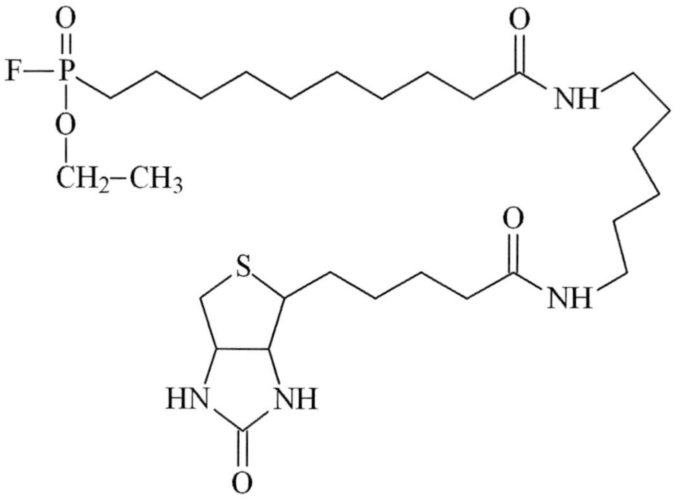

Figure 7.The structure of FP-biotin.

The nerve agents soman and sarin were shown to bind covalently to a tyrosine residue of HSA (Black *et al.*, 1999; Adams *et al.*, 2004). The treatment of the covalently modified albumin with potassium fluoride results in the release of the nerve agents (Adams *et al.*, 2004). Finally, MALDI-TOF mass spectrometry provided direct evidence that the organophosphates chlorpyrifos oxon, dichlorvos, DFP, sarin (Li *et al.*, 2007) and soman (Li *et al.*, 2008) were attached to Tyr-411 of human albumin. The organophosphorus compounds sarin, soman, cyclosarin and tabun also phosphylate a tyrosine residue on albumin in human blood (Williams *et al.*, 2007). Adducts of the compounds with albumin are relatively stable and are not degraded by the therapy with oximes. These characteristics make them able to be used as relatively long-lived biological markers of nerve agent exposure. Adducts of all four nerve agents were detected in the blood of exposed guinea pigs in studies for the improvement of medical countermeasures. The tyrosine adducts with soman and tabun were detected in guinea pigs, which received therapy for 7 days after subcutaneous administration of five times the LD50 dose of the respective nerve agent. Mass spectrometric analysis of trypsin hydrolysate of sarin- and soman-modified albumin fraction of blood serum demonstrated that the modified tyrosine residue resided within peptide 411-Tyr-Thr-Lys-413 (Williams *et al.*, 2007).

Tyr-411 is the most reactive amino acid residue in reaction with phosphoroorganic compounds, though some other residues also are subjected to modification. Indeed, the authors (Means and Wu, 1979) showed that upon HSA interaction with diisopropylfluorophosphate, only up to 90% of the protein contained modified Tyr-411. The remaining 10% of the protein molecules were modified at some other amino acid residues. Using LC-ESI mass spectrometry, Black and coauthors (Black *et al.*, 1999) demonstrated that incubation of human serum with sarin and subsequent pronase hydrolysis of the serum proteins results in the appearance in the mass spectrum of protonated molecular ions corresponding to *O*-isopropylmethylphosphonylserine and *O*-isopropylmethylphosphonyl tyrosine. Similar molecular ions corresponding to serine and tyrosine derivatives were revealed after serum incubation with soman (Black *et al.*, 1999), cyclosarin and tabun (Williams *et al.*, 2007). A second site for covalent attachment of soman was also suggested from the observations that more amounts of fluoride ion was released than could be accounted for by one site in albumin (Li *et al.*, 2008). Pre-treatment of albumin with decanoate, a lipid that binds to the Tyr-411-containing subdomain, inhibited the incorporation of 91% of the ^{3}H-DFP, while the other 9% of the ^{3}H-DFP was possibly bound to other sites (Means and Wu, 1979).

The authors (Ding *et al.*, 2008) investigated the hypothesis that other residues in albumin could be modified by organophosphorus agents. Human plasma was aggressively treated with FP-biotin (Figure 7); plasma proteins were separated into high and low abundant portions using a proteome partitioning antibody kit, and the proteins were digested with trypsin. The FP-biotinylated tryptic peptides were isolated by binding to monomeric avidin beads. The major sites of covalent attachment identified by mass spectrometry were Tyr-138, Tyr-148, Tyr-401, Tyr-411, Tyr-452, Syr-232 and Ser-287 of human albumin. Prolonged treatment of pure human albumin with chlorpyrifos oxon labeled Tyr-138, Tyr-150, Tyr-161, Tyr-401, Tyr-411 and Tyr-452. Therefore, it was shown that, along with Tyr-411, five tyrosines and two serines in human albumin are labeled by the organophosphorus agent FP-biotin (Ding *et al.*, 2008).

Although enantioselectivity was observed for several substrates, Li and co-authors (Li *et al.*, 2008) showed by ^{31}P NMR spectroscopy and computer modeling that human serum albumin interacted with four soman stereoisomers with the same efficiency (rate constant of phosphonylation was found to be 15 ± 3 $M^{-1}min^{-1}$). Rate constant of spontaneous HSA regeneration at pH 8.0 and 25 °C was 4.4×10^{-3} h^{-1} ($\tau_{1/2} = 6.5$ days). Stability of phosphonylated albumin increasedat pH 7.4 and 22 °C ($\tau_{1/2} = 20$ days). Though the concentration of albumin in plasma is very high (about 0.6 mM), its reactivity with organophosphates (phosphonylation and phosphotriesterase activity) is too slow to play a major role in the detoxification of the highly toxic compounds.

Serum albumin is also capable of hydrolyzing carbaryl (1-naphtyl-*N*-methylcarbamate) and 4-nitrophenyl *N*-methylcarbamate (Kuhr and Dorough, 1976; Sogorb *et al.*, 2002; Sogorb *et al.*, 2004). The carbaryl-hydrolyzing activity of HSA was previously described by Casida and Augustinsson (Casida and Augustinsson, 1959a). The activity was demonstrated to be specific toward the studied substrates, since serum albumins were not able to hydrolyze carbamyl cholines or *N,N*-dimethylcarbamyl fluoride (Casida and Augustinsson, 1959b; Kuhr and Dorough, 1976). Carboxylesterase activities associated with albumin were variable among species. Among albumins investigated, the maximal hydrolytic efficiency was observed in the presence of rabbit serum albumin (Sogorb *et al.*, 2002), a bit less active were found to be human and bovine albumins and the least activity was found for chicken serum protein (Sogorb *et al.*, 2002). The kinetic parameters for the product (1-naphtol) formation were determined to be $k_{cat} = 7{,}1\times10^{-5}$ s^{-1} and $K_m = 240$ μM (Sogorb *et al.*, 2002). Carborylase activity of rabbit serum albumin was inhibited by 50% by Cu^{2+} (1mM) and was not affected by Ca^{2+}, Zn^{2+}, Mg^{2+}, Mn^{2+}, Na^{+}, K^{+} and EDTA (5 mM) (Sogorb *et al.*, 2002). At the same time, the catalytic activity of HSA was slightly higher in the presence of Zn^{2+}, Mn^{2+}, Cd^{2+}, Ni^{2+}, Na^{+} (1 mM) and 0.01 mM Pb^{2+} (Sogorb *et al.*, 2004).

The authors (Sogorb *et al.*, 2002; Sogorb *et al.*, 2004) used selective amino acid reagents, specific inhibitors and other competitive substrates to conclude that HSA and RSA hydrolyze carbaryl through the transient reversible carbamylation of the Tyr-411 residue of both albumins. The proposed mechanism for the hydrolysis of carbaryl by HSA is displayed in Scheme 9. This mechanism might be based on the initial carbamylation of Tyr-411 of HSA in the sequence Arg-Tyr-Thr-Arg. Thecarbamylation would cause the release of 1-naphthol and yield a carbamylated Tyr residue. This Tyr could be further decarbamylated through the nucleophilic attack of a water molecule yielding free enzyme and carbamic acid. The released carbamic acid instantaneously decomposes into CO_2 and methylamine. This mechanism is similar to the mechanism described for serine esterases (like acetylcholinesterase), but with tyrosine instead of serine playing the most important role. The specific carbarylase activity of human serum was around six times lower than the same activity of HSA (Sogorb *et al.*, 2004). This can be explained by the inhibitory effects of fatty acids. Despite the lower activity of albumin as a part of serum, the protein can still be considered a detoxification system, since its efficacy in this process is based on the extraordinary large number of the protein molecules. Indeed, serum albumin represents more than 50% of total protein in serum (Peters, 1996), and because the inhibition by fatty acids is not complete, this suggests the presence of a number of molecules with the capability to hydrolyze carbaryl. In addition, the contribution of albumins to carbamate detoxification must not be considered only in serum because serum contains only around 30% of the total albumin amount in the whole animal body (Peters, 1996). These extravascular molecules of albumin possess different affinity to fatty acids depending on the tissue (gut, liver, muscle, or skin). Finally, all albumin present in the body is synthesized in the liver (Peters, 1996), and this protein is synthesized fatty acid-free. The liver is an important reservoir of active detoxifying protein and probably is the most important organ involved in the hydrolysis of carbamates by albumins (Sogorb *et al.*, 2002; Sogorb *et al.*, 2004). The hydrolysis of carbaryl by BSA was studied at toxicologically-relevant concentrations (range 15-300 μM) in order to determine the role of this protein in the detoxification of carbamates *in vivo* (Sogorb *et al.*, 2007). The estimated turnover and Michaelis-Menten constant were calculated to be $1.6\times10^{-4}s^{-1}$ and 430 μM, respectively. Thus, the second order rate constant was 0.37 $M^{-1}s^{-1}$.At enzyme concentrations of 7.0 mg ml^{-1} and the substrate concentrations ranging between 50 and 300 μM, about 80% of the substrate was hydrolyzed in 3 h. Significant hydrolysis was detected even at lower carbaryl concentrations (15 and 30 μM). Although the efficacy of the enzymatic hydrolysis is low, the extrapolation of these results to the physiological albumin's concentration (around 40 mg ml^{-1}) suggests that the hydrolysis of carbaryl by serum albumins plays a critical role in the detoxification of this carbamate at *in vivo* toxicologically-relevant concentrations. The knowledge of the chemical structure-activity relationship of the carbamate-hydrolyzing activity associated with serum albumins could be very important for the assessment of risk of the carbamate insecticides to humans. An ideal insecticide should be active against insects, while its activity in vertebrates, who possess albumin, should be abolished due to the protein's action.

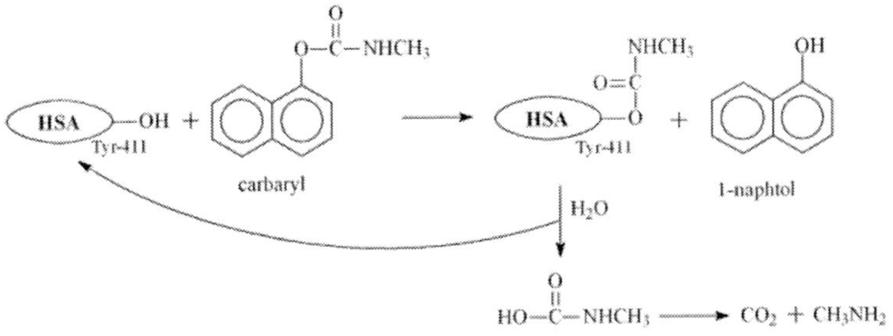

Scheme 9.

Nicotinate esters were studied in terms of their binding and hydrolysis by HSA (Steiner *et al.*, 1992; Salvi *et al.*, 1997). It was observed that the hydrolysis efficiency depended on the alcohol structure and was determined by both electronic and spatial factors. The hydrolysis rate for *n*-alkyl esters (methyl, ethyl, *n*-propyl, *n*-butyl, and *n*-hexyl nicotinate esters) increased with the increase in the number of methylene elements in alkyl radical. Thus, 1 mg HSA hydrolyzed 0.53 μmoles of *n*-butyl ester of nicotinic acid per minute, whereas for methyl ester, only 0.0188 min required to hydrolyze the same amount of the substrate. In contrast to non-enzymatic hydrolysis (Wernly-Chung *et al.*, 1990), steric hindrance reduced the rate of albumin-catalyzed hydrolysis, as seen upon comparison of the correspondent rate constants for *n*-butyl, isobutyl and *tert*-butyl nicotinate esters. For instance, the rate constant for the hydrolysis of isobutyl ester of nicotinic acid is twice as low as that for the correspondent *n*-butyl ester (2.9×10^{-3} and 5.6×10^{-3} min^{-1}, respectively). The two amides investigated, namely carbamoylmethyl and 1-carbamoylethyl nicotinate, were very poor substrates, the latter being even stabilized against hydrolysis by the presence of HSA. Maximal efficiency of albumin-catalyzed hydrolysis was observed for 2-butoxyethyl and 2-(*N,N*-diethylamino)-ethyl esters of nicotinic acid ($k = 5.04 \times 10^{-2}$ min^{-1} and 4.1×10^{-2} min^{-1},respectively; pH 7.40 ± 0.10, 37 °C± 0.2 °C).

It was observed that a component of human serum could trigger the release of mercaptoethanol from *S*-lauroylmercaptoethanol (S-LME) (Kurooka and Yoshimura, 1973). Efficiency of the substrate hydrolysis was the same for the serum and the purified albumin. This finding allowed the authors to conclude that HSA was the main thioesterase that catalyzed *S*-lauroylmercaptoethanol hydrolysis in blood. The mercaptoethanol-releasing activity was also found in serum albumins from other mammals, but not in ovalbumin. Among *S*-C_{10}, *S*-C_{12}, *S*-C_{14}, and *S*-C_{16} acylmercaptoethanols tested at pH 8.0, *S*-lauroylmercaptoethanol was the best substrate, whereas *O*-acetyl-*S*- lauroylmercaptoethanol was not hydrolyzed at all, suggesting that the OH group of *S*-lauroylmercaptoethanol is necessary for the interaction. Maximal cleavage efficiency was observed at pH 9-10. The activity was diminished greatly after about 8 moles of mercaptoethanol had been released per one mole of HSA. The mercaptoethanol-releasing activity was practically absent in acidic medium. In addition, the activity was completely lost when HSA was acetylated by acetic anhydride or *N*-acetylimidazole, or maleylated with maleic anhydride. Therefore, the authors (Kurooka and Yoshimura, 1973) concluded that *S*-lauroylmercaptoethanol hydrolysis in the presence of serum albumin proceeded via acetylation of the protein's lysine residues and, less probably, serine residues (Scheme 10). The mercaptoethanol-releasing reaction is specific for albumin. This activity can be applied for the assay to measure serum or urinary albumins.

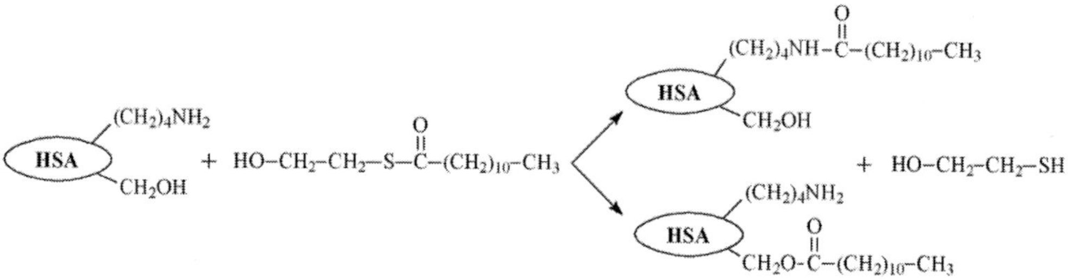

Scheme 10.

Albumin is also able to act as a thioesterase due to the presence of a free sulfhydryl group at Cys-34. For example, the protein can degrade tetraethylthiuram disulfide (disulfiram), which is a clinically important reaction (Agarwal *et al.*, 1986). The efficiency of disulfiram (Antabuse) as a drug used for the treatment of alcohol abuse is limited by the fact that it is degraded rapidly in the tissues and in the serum. The authors (Agarwal *et al.*, 1986) have reported that degradation of disulfiram in serum results from a covalent interaction of the drug with the free sulfhydryl group of serum albumin (Scheme 11). At pH 9, the half-time for this process was 30-40 s, while at pH 7.4, the reaction rate was decreased (the half-time was 1-1.5 min). These results suggest that degradation of disulfiram by serum albumin is physiologically and clinically important, since the drug becomes maximally active only many hours after administration.

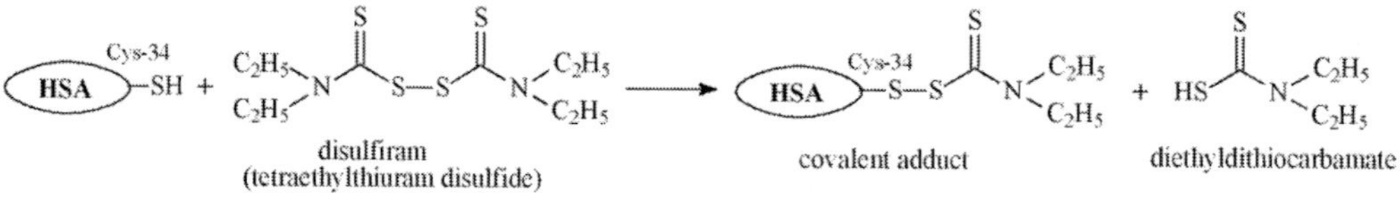

Scheme 11.

Summary. Serum albumin seems to play important pharmacokinetic and physiological roles not only by binding and transporting drugs and endogenous compounds, but also by acting as a pseudo-esterase. In other words, serum albumin contains both binding and catalytic sites. HSA appears to have one markedly reactive site (Kurono *et al.*, 1992) and multiple non-specific catalytic sites (Means and Bender, 1975). Tyr-411, Lys-199 and Arg-410 are essential for the pseudo-esterase activity of HSA.

2.1.3. *β-Lactamase Activity of Serum Albumin*

β-Lactam antibiotics feature a five-membered thiazolidine ring fused to a four-membered *β*-lactam ring. The latter ring is strained. It includes an amide moiety that has a critical role in the inactivation of the synthesis of peptidoglycan, which is the major component of the rigid cell wall protecting bacteria from osmotic lysis. When penicillin binds to transpeptidase, an active-site Ser attacks the carbonyl of the *β*-lactam ring and generates a covalent adduct between penicillin and the enzyme. However, the leaving group remains attached to the enzyme because it is linked by the remnant of the *β*-lactam ring (Figure 8). The covalent complex irreversibly inactivates the enzyme. This, in turn, blocks the synthesis of the bacterial cell wall, and most bacteria die as the fragile inner membrane bursts under osmotic pressure.

The plasma proteins have been reported to exert irreversible effects on some *β*-lactam antibiotics (Bruderleun *et al.*, 1981). The human plasma proteins were fractionated on a Sephadex column and the fractions were tested individually. The albumin's fraction was found to be entirely responsible for the destruction, while the globulin's fraction was completely inactive. Displacement of a fluorescent probe (5-dimethylaminonaphthalene-1-sulfoamide) by (+/-)-2-methylpenem-3-carboxylic acid (a prototype of *β*-lactam antibiotic) showed that the binding site for the latter is the same as the one occupied by L-tryptophan. Lysine residues are involved in the albumin-catalyzed penicillins destruction.

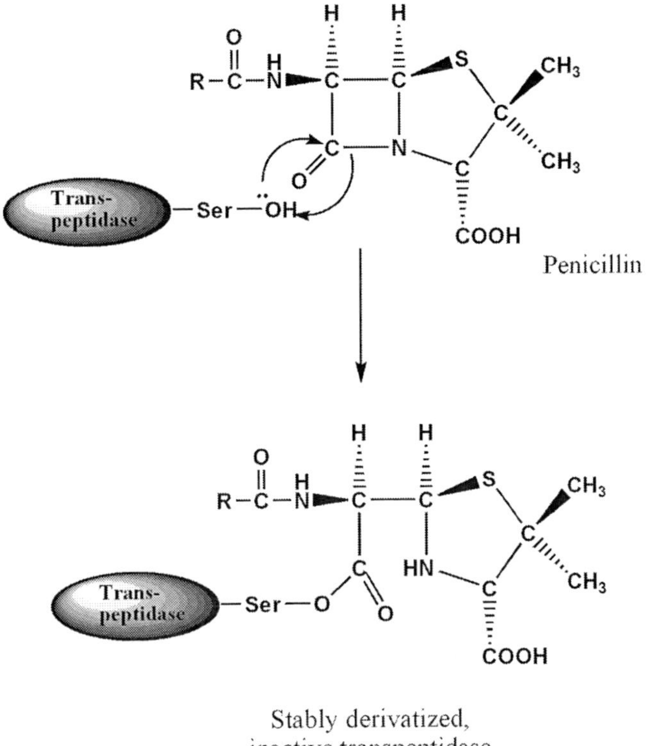

Figure 8.Transpeptidase inhibition by *β*-lactam antibiotics. Attack on the amide moiety of the *β*-lactam ring by a transpeptidase active-site Ser results in a covalent acyl-enzyme product. The covalent adduct is hydrolyzed so slowly that its formation is practically irreversible, and the transpeptidase is inactivated.

The principal mode of albumin's interaction with penicillins involves the formation of amide bonds through an aminolysis reaction with lysine groups of HSA (Díaz *et al.*, 2001b).

The resulting adduct has an opened β-lactam ring (penicilloyl group), which has no antibacterial activity (Levine and Ovary, 1961) (Scheme 12).

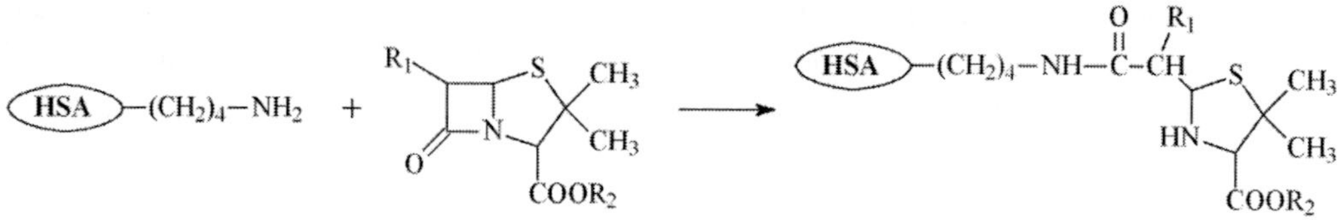

Scheme 12.

The primary site of penicilloyl coupling is the ε-amino group of Lys-199, though penicilloyl groups have been also detected experimentally on other lysine residues of HSA (Lys-190, Lys-195, Lys-432, Lys-541, and Lys-545) (Yvon *et al.*, 1988; Yvon *et al.*, 1989; Yvon *et al.*, 1990). Interestingly, Lys-195 is near Lys-199 in the subdomain IIA binding site (site I), suggesting that the combination of two closely located ε-amino groups could have possible structural and/or mechanistic consequences. In the case of site I, molecular dynamics simulations have shown that the most likely configuration for the Lys-195/Lys-199 pair corresponds to the neutral ε-amino group of Lys-199 connected to the acid form of Lys-195 through a network of H-bonding water molecules (Díaz *et al.*, 2001a). The authors (Díaz *et al.*, 2001b) have proposed that this acid-base pair could undergo proton interchange easily and, consequently, both lysine residues could have an enhanced nucleophilic ability, as experimentally observed in the case of penicillin binding to HSA (Yvon *et al.*, 1988; Yvon *et al.*, 1989; Yvon *et al.*, 1990). These authors note that similar considerations could apply to the other two penicillin binding sites. It ispossible that each pair of lysine residues constitutes an acid-base pair subjected to water-assisted proton interchange so that the lone pair of the neutral amino group could be a more effective nucleophile against penicillins (Díaz *et al.*, 2001b). Furthermore, X-ray structure of HSA (Sugio *et al.*, 1999) has also revealed that the pairing of lysine residues (e.g. Lys190/Lys-432 and Lys541/Lys545) is a major feature of other penicillin binding sites. This structural pairing of the reactive lysine groups is consistent with the experimental observation that there are never more than two or three penicillin molecules bound to a single HSA molecule (Fischer and Jardeztky, 1965).

It was found that albumin of different purity obtained from a variety of sources, showed a significant β-lactamase activity (Nerli and Picó, 1994; Nerli *et al.*, 1995). Purified albumin was shownto have a hydrolase activity, catalyzing the decomposition of the chromogenic cephalosporin: 3-(2,4-dinitrostyryl)-(6R, 7R)-7-(2-thienacetamodo)-ceph-3-em-4-carboxylic acid (nitrocefin). The reaction demonstrated saturation kinetics with a K_m of 1.42×10^{-5} M. Oleic acid and ibuprofen inhibited the reaction, suggesting that the cephalosporin and these ligands are bound to the same site of albumin (Nerli and Picó, 1994; Nerli *et al.*, 1995). The binding to HSA of some cephalosporins of pharmacological interest was studied using an ultrafiltration method (Nerli *et al.*, 1997). Cephalosporins were classified into three groups according to their affinity for albumin: low affinity (K = 10-10^2 M^{-1}), medium affinity (K = 10^3 M^{-1}) and high affinity (K = 10^4 M^{-1}). Cephalosporin binding to albumin produced a perturbation of several basic amino acids of the protein such as histidine and lysine. It was found that only cefuroxime, ceftazidime and cefoperazone interacted slightly with site I on serum albumin, while site II possessed the capacity to bind cephradine, cephalexin, ceftazidime, ceftriaxone, cefoperazone, cefaclor and cefsulodin. The binding sites for cephalosporins on albumin are structurally heterogenic, having different amino acids in the vicinity of the ligand molecule. Cephalosporins interact with HSA at the binding regions that involve Tyr-411, His-146, Lys-195, Lys-199, Lys-225, Lys-240 and Lys-525. The authors (Nerli and Picó, 1994) suggested that the tertiary structure of albumin is necessary for the catalytic activity. The dimeric and trimeric form of albumin also possessed this hydrolase activity (Nerli *et al.*, 1995).

It was demonstrated that HSA showed a stereoselective binding and degradation of sulbencillin isomers (Tsuda *et al.*, 2001). Using site-specific markers, it was revealed that site I (warfarin binding site) preferentially bound *R*-sulbencillin isomer: the binding constant for *R*-isomer was approximately 2.3-fold greater than that of *S*-isomer. The same stereoselectivity was observed for sulbencillin degradation. Indeed, the degradation rate constant for *R*-sulbencillin was approximately 7-fold greater than that for *S*-sulbencillin.The results demonstrate that site I might be responsible for the stereoselective degradation of sulbencillin.

An attack on the amide moiety of the β-lactam ring by the albumin's Lys residues results in a covalent acyl-protein product. This is hydrolyzed so slowly that adduct formation is practically irreversible. Therefore, penicilloyl-albumin conjugates are accumulated. Most importantly, these penicilloyl-albumin complexes, which have lost all antibacterial activity, constitute the major antigenic determinant of penicillin allergy (Levine and Ovary, 1961; Saxon *et al.*, 1987).

2.2. Serum Albumin as a Lyase and Isomerase

Serum albumin was found to possess enolase-like activity towards dihydrotestosterone, converting its 3-keto to 3-enol form (Drmanovic *et al.*, 1999) (Scheme 13).

Enolase-like activity was found in serum of all mammalian species studied, though the specific activity was very low in the serum of dogs. In addition to serum albumin, enolase-like activity was found to be a feature of intracellular albumin. The two albumins exhibited the same specific activity and the same K_m for dihydrotestosterone. The administration of dihydrotestosterone in mice did not influence the level of albumin or its enolase activity in their serum. The activity was strongly inhibited by Ni (II) and Cu (II) ions, which were bound to a histidine residue of the albumin molecule, as well as by oleic acid and cholesterol. The activity was also inhibited, in a reversible manner, by surface-active agents. The enolase-like activity of HSA is influenced by pH and the type of the buffer used (Drmanovic *et al.*, 1999; Matsushita *et al.*, 2004).

The maximal enolase activity of albumin was observed at pH 9.2 in a carbonate buffer solution. The authors (Matsushita *et al.*, 2004) used *Pichia pastoris* to separately express the three recombinant domains of HSA, in order to determine the location of the catalytic sites for albumin's enolase-like activity. All domains showed a decrease in enolase-like activity at pH 7.4 in the phosphate buffer, with domain II showing the lowest value, compared with rHSA. In contrast, all domains and rHSA showed an increase in activity at pH 9.2 in the carbonate buffer. Among the domains, domain II showed the largest increase, suggesting that an enolase catalytic site is generated in domain II upon pH alteration(Matsushita *et al.*, 2004).

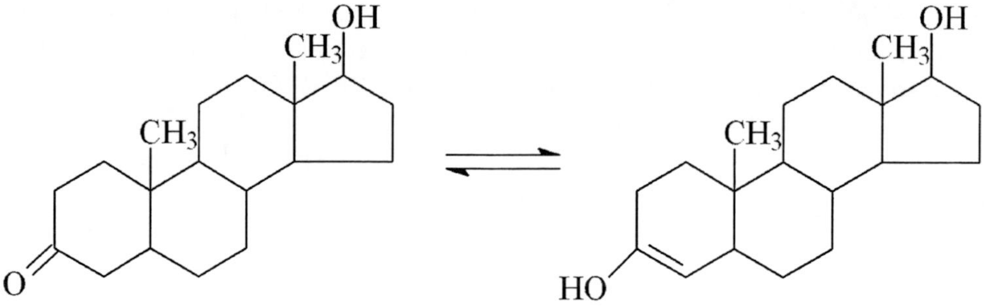

Scheme 13.

The enolase-like activity of HSA can be of clinical use. Intracellular accumulation of albumin has been observed in the cytosol of benign and malignant human breast tumors and in mammary tumors of rodents induced by carcinogens (Bhat *et al.*, 1998). Cells of benign breast tumors have a much higher concentration of cytosolic albumin, which allows differentiating this tumor type from the malignant breast tumors. In addition, the intrinsic enolase-like activity of both serum and cytosolic HSA is much lower in cytosol from malignant tumors. The reduced activity is partly due to the lower albumin concentration and partly due to polymerization and/or binding of the protein to other intracellular proteins. Taken together, these two parameters (intracellular albumin's concentration and its enolase activity) provide a basis for reliable differentiation between benign and malignant breast tumors (Drmanovic *et al.*, 1999).

Albumin seems to have a significant role in both the elimination and biosynthesis of prostaglandin D_2 (PGD_2) (Watanabe *et al.*, 1982). PGD_2 is formed in a variety of tissues and cells and modulates their functions under various physiological and pathological conditions. A potential anti-neoplastic effect of PGD_2 has been reported (Fukushima *et al.*, 1982a). It has been found that 9-deoxy-Δ^9-PGD_2, a dehydration product of PGD_2, has about three times stronger growth inhibitory effect on L-1210 leukemia cultured cells than PGD_2 (Fukushima *et al.*, 1982b).

The authors (Kikawa *et al.*, 1984) reported the conversion of PGD_2 in human plasma to a compound that was identified as 9-deoxy-9,10-didehydro-12,13-didehydro-13,14-dihydro-PGD_2 (9-deoxy-$\Delta^{9,12}$-13,14-dihydro-PGD_2). Similar conversion was also demonstrated upon incubation of PGD_2 with HSA at the protein's concentration equal to that found in plasma. These results suggest that the formation of 9-deoxy-$\Delta^{9,12}$-13,14-dihydro-PGD_2 in dialyzed plasma is catalyzed by serum albumin itself.

The authors (Fitzpatrick and Wynalda, 1981) determined the effect of vertebrate albumins on the stability of several physiologically relevant prostaglandins. For all naturally occurring prostaglandins with β-hydroxy ketone group, first-order kinetics for concentration-dependent albumin-catalyzed decomposition was observed in 0.1 M, pH 7.4 buffer at 37 °C. Albumin had no destructive effect on prostaglandins without a β-hydroxy ketone group. Later, these authors (Fitzpatrick and Wynalda, 1983) determined the structures of three products that originated from albumin-catalyzed transformation of prostaglandin D_2 (PGD_2), namely 9-deoxy-11-keto-15α-hydroxy-$\Delta^{5,9,12}$-prostenoic acid (9-deoxy-$\Delta^{9,12}$-PGD_2); 15-deoxy-11-keto-9α-hydroxy-$\Delta^{5,12,14}$-prostenoic acid (15-deoxy-$\Delta^{12,14}$-PGD_2); and 9,15-dideoxy-11-keto-$\Delta^{5,9,12,14}$-prostenoic acid (9,15-dideoxy-$\Delta^{9,12,14}$-PGD_2 (Scheme 14).

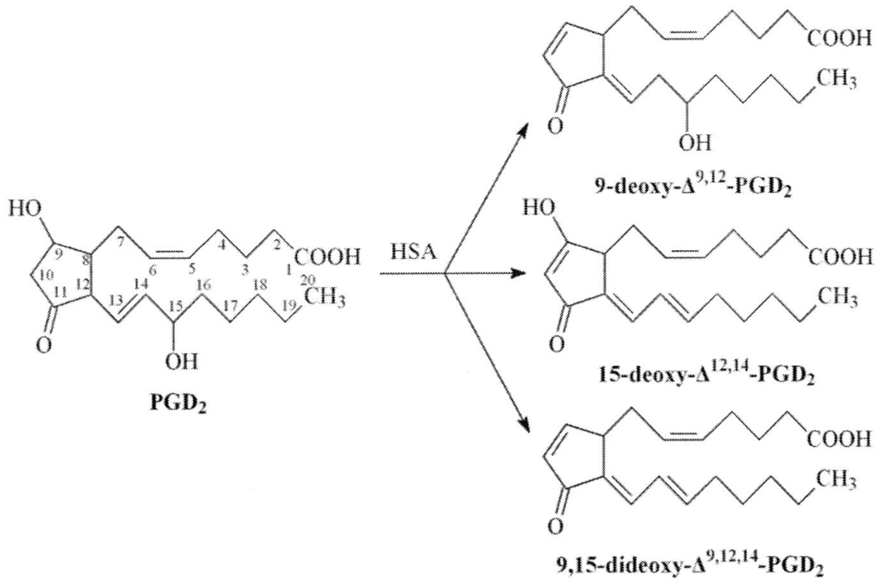

Scheme 14.

The results suggest that albumin sequesters prostaglandins in one principal binding site and exposes them to its highly alkaline microenvironment. Prostaglandin D_2 contains a proton at C_{12} that is simultaneously allylic and in the α-position to the carbonyl group. Therefore, even mildly alkaline conditions facilitate isomerization of the *β,γ*-unsaturated enone to a more stable *α,β*-unsaturated enone. Isomerization of the lower side chain olefin occurs so readily that the synthesis of ring-dehydrated isomers directly from PGD_2 is impossible without concurrent Δ^{12}-isomer formation (Bundy *et al.*, 1983). It is likely that Δ^{12}-isomerization facilitates dehydration of the C_{15} hydroxyl. The biochemical significance of these results is uncertain. PGD_2*in vivo* is inactivated by different metabolic processes than those typical for other prostaglandins. Rather than widely distributed NAD-linked dehydrogenases, organ-specific NAD-linked dehydrogenase (Tokumoto *et al.*, 1982) and 11-keto-reductase (Ellis *et al.*, 1979) dominate the metabolism of PGD_2. Fitzpatrick andWynalda suggested that albumin-catalyzed transformation of PGD_2 could also occur *in vivo* as a supplementary inactivation process (Fitzpatrick and Wynalda, 1983).

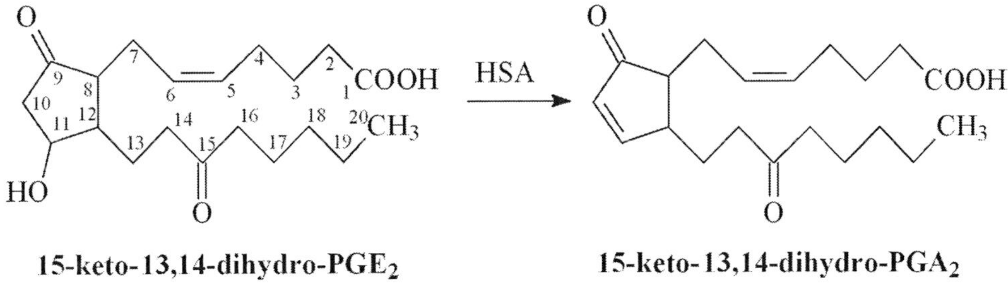

Scheme 15.

In samples containing albumin, 15-keto-dihydro-PGE_2 was degraded more rapidly than in a buffer of the same pH (Granström *et al.*, 1980). In addition to the formation of the dehydration products, a considerable part of the metabolite was bound to albumin to yield water soluble adducts. A similar binding occurred to a low molecular weight fraction of plasma. The compound that was bound was 15-keto-dihydro-PGA_2 (Scheme 15), whereas both 15-keto-dihydro-PGE_2 and the bicyclic product were relatively inert in this respect.

Several authors (Hamberg and Fredholm, 1976; Watanabe *et al.*, 1982) have shown that in the presence of serum albumin from a number of species, prostaglandin H_2 decomposes mainly into prostaglandin D_2, an isomer of prostaglandin E_2 (Scheme 16A). The optimal pH and K_m value for prostaglandin H_2 were 9.0 and 6 μM, respectively. This albumin's activity under physiological conditions was examined in a model system constituted of serum albumin and washed platelets (Watanabe *et al.*, 1982). Prostaglandin D_2 formation was observed in association with thrombin-evoked platelet aggregation in this system. The amount of PGD_2 formed was proportional to the number of platelets and the concentration of serum albumin. The data allowed the authors to suggest that thrombin-stimulated platelets released prostaglandin H_2, which was then converted to prostaglandin D_2 by the action of serum albumin. This interpretation was supported by the following observation: prostaglandin H_2 added to platelet-rich plasma was converted in part to prostaglandin D_2. In aqueous solutions, the prostaglandin endoperoxide PGH_2 decomposes mainly into prostaglandin E_2 (Scheme 16B) (Hamberg and Fredholm, 1976). Taking into account that prostaglandins can be released from tissues into the bloodstream, the authors (Hamberg and Fredholm, 1976) suggested that the effect of serum albumin on endoperoxide decomposition may have physiological significance. Indeed, albumin-catalyzed PGH_2 transformation results in PGD_2, which biological properties are quite different from the properties of PGE_2.

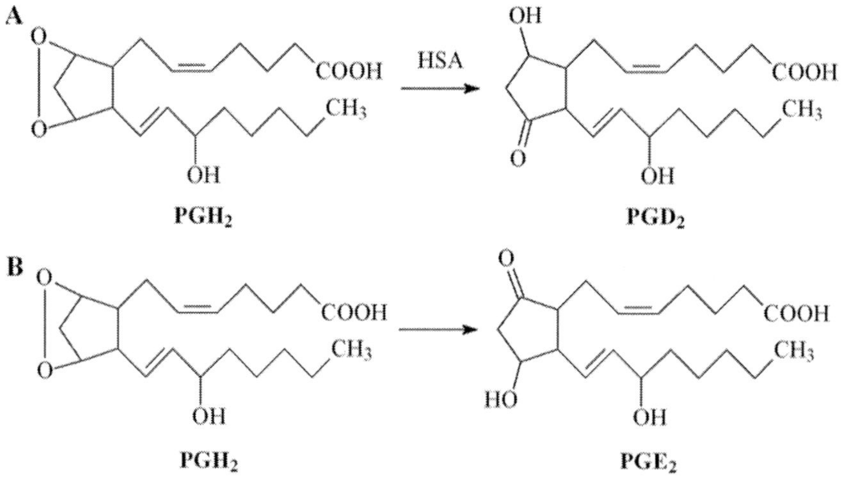

Scheme 16.

HSA has been shown to display some limited lyase activity with drug metabolites such as felbamate (Roller *et al.*, 2002) and 4-hydroxycyclophosphamide (Kwon *et al.*, 1987).

Cyclophosphamide, which was first discovered about forty years ago, is one of the most successful anti-cancer drugs developed over the last few decades. It is effective against a variety of human cancers. In the body, cyclophosphamide is activated by cytochrome P-450

(CYP450) in the liver, which results in the release of activated phosphoramide mustard and acrolein (Kwon *et al.*, 1987) (Scheme 17). As shown in Scheme 17, (CYP450) converts cyclophosphamide to 4-hydroxycyclophosphamide, which undergoes ring opening to form aldophosphamide. The latter is then converted into a phosphoramide mustard and acrolein via base-catalyzed β-elimination. Phosphoramide mustard is the final alkylating agent responsible for cross-linking DNA strands, which leads to cell death.

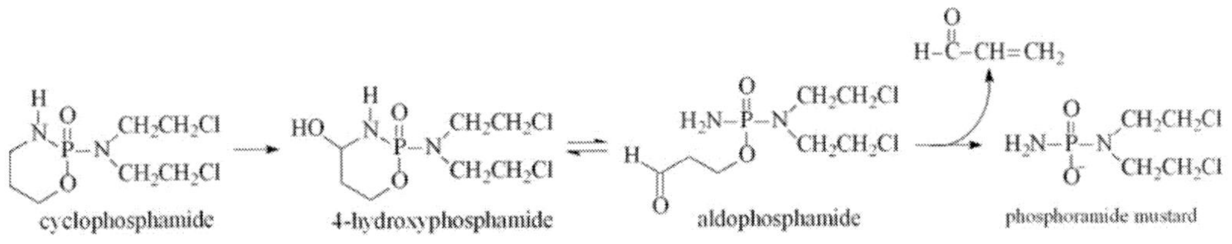

Scheme 17.

Serum albumin was identified as a catalyst for the elimination step, whichgeneratedphosphoramide mustard from aldolphosphamide. The rate of ring opening of 4-hydroxycyclophosphamide to yield aldophosphamide was not affected by the protein. The catalytic activity of serum albumin was dependent on the protein's concentration and independent of pH over the range of 6.5 to 7.5, in contrast to the buffer-catalyzed reaction. The catalytic rate constants k_{cat} (pH 7.4, 37 ^{0}C) for phosphate buffer, HSA, and BSA were 1.13 min^{-1}M^{-1}, 285 min^{-1}M^{-1}, and 83 min^{-1}M^{-1}, respectively.

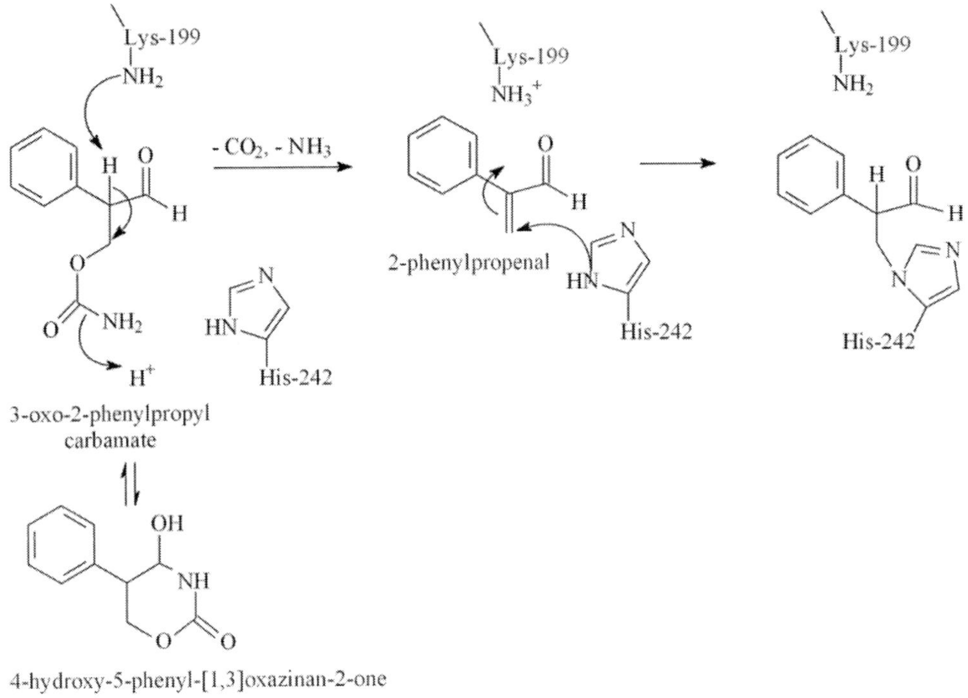

Scheme 18.

Serum albumin also catalyzes one of the metabolic steps for an anti-epileptic drug felbamate. Felbamate (2-phenyl-1,3-propanediol dicarbamate) is associated with hepatotoxicity (O'Nell *et al.*, 1996) and aplastic anemia (Pennell *et al.*, 1995). The toxicities are believed to be caused by the formation of 2-phenylpropenal, a highly reactive felbamate metabolite. The authors (Roller *et al.*, 2002) have demonstrated that felbamate is metabolized into 3-oxo-2-phenylpropyl carbamate. Under physiological conditions, the metabolite undergoes β-elimination to form the α,β-unsaturated aldehyde 2-phenylpropenal. At the same time, 3-oxo-2-phenylpropyl carbamate exists in equilibrium with 4-hydroxy-5-phenyl-[1,3]oxazinan-2-one (Scheme 18).

It was demonstrated that the half-life of the oxazinane at pH 7.4 is greatly reduced in the presence of HSA when compared to an aqueous buffer (Dieckhaus *et al.*, 2001). The HSA-catalyzed decomposition of the oxazinane was found to have a k_{cat} of 12.04 $min^{-1}M^{-1}$. This k_{cat} is an order of magnitude lower than the k_{cat} for the HSA-catalyzed decomposition of the structurally similar molecule 4-hydroxycyclophosphamide (k_{cat} = 285 $min^{-1}M^{-1}$) (Kwon *et al.*, 1987) and about the same as for the HSA-catalyzed β-elimination of various prostaglandins (k_{cat} ranges from ~1 to 21 $min^{-1}M^{-1}$, as calculated by Roller (Roller *et al.*, 2002) using data reported by Fitzpatrick and Wynalda (Fitzpatrick and Wynalda, 1981)).

According to the data on competitive binding assays with warfarin and ibuprofen, HSA-catalyzed decomposition of the oxazinane involves the subdomain IIA binding site of HSA (Roller *et al.*, 2002). As mentioned earlier, subdomain IIA is known to be involved in the hydrolysis of several small molecules, such as aspirin and penicillins, through nucleophilic attack by Lys-199. In these examples, Lys-199 is covalently modified at the ε-amino group. LC/MS/MS analyses of trypsin digests of HSA incubated with the oxazinane or 2-phenylpropenal identified that amino acid residues His-242 and His-247 are the sites for HSA-2-phenylpropenal adducts formation. While 2-phenylpropenal does not alkylate Lys-199, the authors (Roller *et al.*, 2002) considered that Lys -199 may act as the basic residue that catalyzes the β-elimination and leads to the decomposition of the oxazinane (Scheme 18). The same idea has been proposed for the HSA-mediated β-elimination of several prostaglandins (Fitzpatrick *et al.*, 1984).

According to the suggested mechanism, the oxazinane is bound to HSA in subdomain IIA in the vicinity of Lys-199. Lys-199 then acts as a general base to deprotonate the oxazinane at the benzyllic position. 2-Phenylpropenal, which is generated by the subsequent β-elimination, can then alkylate the neighboring His-242 or His-247 residues. The formation of these HSA-2-phenylpropenal adducts are reversible. The alkylation extent after extensive dialysis decreases by $74.0 \pm 0.6\%$ (Roller *et al.*, 2002).

Although the k_{cat} for the oxazinane decomposition seems to be small, the HSA-oxazinane interaction may have some significance *in vivo*. Because the physiological concentration of HSA is so high in plasma (~0.6 mM) and the concentration of the oxazinane is relatively low (< 50 μM), the effect on the half-life of the oxazinane is quite dramatic. Under physiological conditions, the half-life of the oxazinane is reduced by over 75%. As a consequence, HSA may contribute considerably to the metabolism of the oxazinane *in vivo* (Roller *et al.*, 2002).

2.3. Serum Albumin as an Oxidoreductase

Lipid peroxidation has been associated with a number of pathophysiological events in a variety of diseases, drug toxicities, traumatic and ischemic injuries. Hence, the prevention of lipid peroxidation is an essential process. A wide array of enzymic and non-enzymic antioxidant defenses exist, including selenium-dependent phospholipids hydroperoxide glutathione peroxidase, glutathione peroxidase, superoxide dismutase, catalase, ascorbic acid, α-tocopherol, glutathione and β-carotene (Halliwell and Gutteridge, 1989). HSA shows antioxidant activity in some assays, and studies have linked the antioxidant activity of HSA to bound bilirubin (Stocker *et al.*, 1987; Stocker and Ames, 1987).Many studies have also indicated an apparent antioxidant role of serum albumin in protection against plasma phospholipids peroxidation (Bao and Williamson, 1996; Cha and Kim, 1996; Hurst *et al.*, 1999; Cha and Kim, 2006). It was found (Bao and Williamson, 1996) that BSA, when used as a carrier in the incorporation of phospholipids hydroperoxide into mammalian cells, results in a slow reduction of the phospholipids hydroperoxide to phospholipids hydroxide. Three years later, Williamson and co-authors (Hurst *et al.*, 1999) have shown that HSA may function as thiol-peroxidase catalyzing reduction of 1-palmitoyl-2-(13-hydroperoxy-*cis*-9,-*trans*-11-octa decaenoyl)-L-3 phosphtidylcholine (PLPC-OOH) to the correspondent hydroxy-derivative (PLPC-OH) (Scheme 19). Although peroxidase activity of the protein towards phosphatidylcholine is observed in the absence of any additional reducing agent, the addition of a thiol-containing co-factor essentially speeds up the albumin-catalyzed reduction reaction. Indeed, the specific activity of HSA (per 1 mg of the protein) is 0.01 nmolemin^{-1} in the absence of co-factors and 0.7 nmolesmin^{-1}, 0.05 nmolesmin^{-1} or 0.02 nmolesmin^{-1} in the presence of cysteine, glutathione or homocysteine as a thiol-containing co-factor, respectively. In the presence of cysteine as a co-factor, the stoichiometric reduction of PLPC-OOH is accompanied by the formation of two cystine molecules.

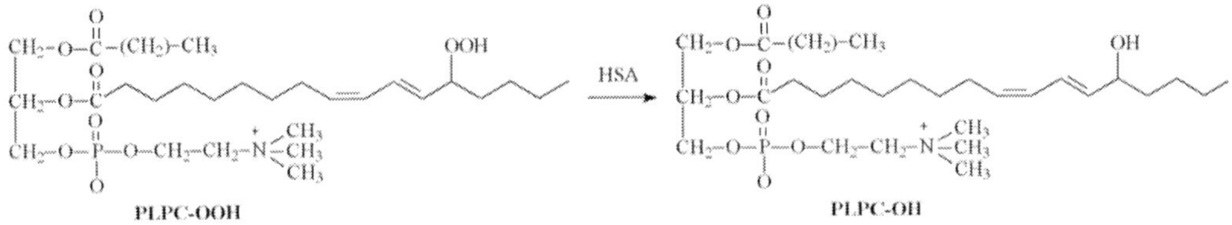

Scheme 19.

The efficiency of phosphatidylcholine peroxide reduction in the presence of HSA is proportionate to the number of free sulfhydryl groups. Thus, modification of Cys-34 SH-group with *N*-ethylmaleimide results in decreasing the peroxidase activity of albumin. Reduction of S-S bridges with DTT enhances the rate of the substrate reduction (Hurst *et al.*, 1999). A similar effect was observed for the interaction of albumin with captopryl, which, in accordance to *Christodoulouet al.* (Christodoulou *et al.*, 1995), deblocks SH-groups implicated in disulfide bonds formation with thiol-containing endogenous substances.In the presence of reduced glutathione, HSA catalyzes decomposition of H_2O_2 (Cha and Kim, 1996). Hydrogen peroxide decomposition is accompanied by the formation of oxidized glutathione. The rate of albumin-catalyzed reaction increases with the protein's concentration reaching saturation. Modification of albumin with reagents specific to sulfhydride groups (*N*-

ethylmaleimide, iodoacetic acid) causes complete inhibition of the protein's peroxidase activity only when modification is carried out in the presence of thiol-containing reductants, such as DTT (Cha and Kim, 1996). This data speaks in favor of the suggestion that cysteine residues involved in the formation of disulfide bridges within HSA molecule participate in the protein's thiolperoxidase activity (Figure 9).

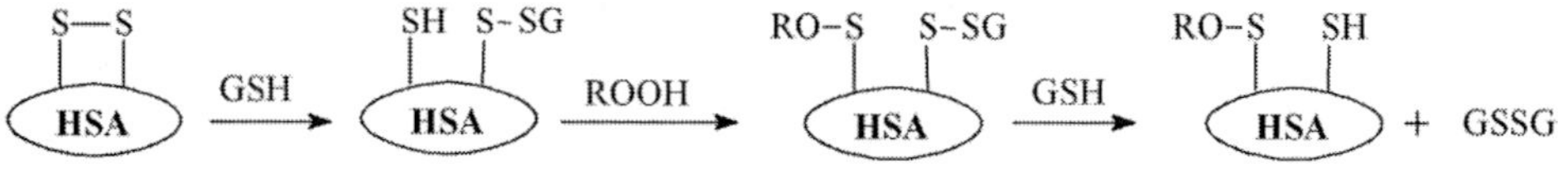

Figure 9.Putative mechanism of peroxide reduction in the presence of HSA with the use of glutathione as an electron donor.

The authors (Cha and Kim, 2006) have revealed that HSA demonstrates an ability to reduce lipid hydroperoxide with the use of thioredoxin as an *in vivo* electron donor. The fragment of the protein-containing domains IIB and III (amino acid residues Pro-299–Leu-585) reduces hydroperoxide of linoleic acid in the presence of thioredoxin more efficiently than the intact protein. The reaction rate is 1.42 ± 0.29pmolemin^{-1}(37 °C) for the protein fragment, in comparison with the value of 0.157 ± 0.010pmolemin^{-1}(30 °C) for the intact protein. Modification of the albumin IIB-III fragment, which had beenreduced with thioredoxin, with a thiol-specific modification agent inactivated the peroxidase activity toward linolic acid peroxide. Mass spectrometric analysis of the tryptic peptides obtained from the inactivated intact albumin or its IIB-III fragment revealed that Cys-392 and Cys-438, which normally form a disulfide bond, were the major modification sites. The obtained data allowed the authors to conclude that the redox-active disulfide bond between Cys-392 and Cys-438 acts as a primary site of the catalysis for the thioredoxin-dependent lipid peroxidase activity of albumin (Cha and Kim, 2006).

The concentration of lipid peroxides is found to increase with age, as well as upon the development of some human diseases including atherosclerosis and Parkinson's disease (Kobayashi *et al.*, 2006). Therefore, a sufficient amount of lipid peroxidase in blood is required to prevent the lipid peroxide-caused diseases. There are many *in vivo* experiments suggesting a lipid peroxidase activity of HSA. For example, it has been demonstrated that analbuminemic rats are more susceptible to oxidative stress than normal rats (Yamamoto *et al.*, 1992). This leads to easier induction of cancers of the urinary bladder, kidney, and stomach by carcinogens. Albumin also inhibites lipid peroxidation in rabbit spermatozoa and protects them against loss of motility (Alvarez and Storey, 1963). HSA decreases the level of peroxidation of erythrocyte membrane lipids (Soejima *et al.*, 1999). Persistent hypoalbuminemia results in the decreased antioxidant activity of serum in chronic hemodialysis patients, which may add to the increased oxidative cell damage (Soejima *et al.*, 1999).

2.4. Unusual Albumin's Catalytic Activities

Several unusual activities were found for serum albumin. One of them is the detoxification of cyanide ions (Jarabak and Westley, 1986). The presence of bovine albumin significantly accelerated the reaction of cyanide ions with colloidal sulfur to form SCN^- ion. The general process may be described by Scheme 20. Reaction rate v_{ss} was found to be described by the shown equation, where [S] is total colloidal sulfur concentration. On the basis of kinetic experiments that measured the effects of a variety of ligands on the sulfur-cyanolysis reaction catalyzed by serum albumin, the authors (Jarabak and Westley, 1989; Jarabak and Westley, 1991) have concluded that the cyanolysis reaction occurs in the protein's subdomain III-AB, near the site occupied by laurate.

Another unusual albumin's activity is its ability to accelerate significantly Meisenheimer complex (1,1-dihydro-2,4,6-trinitrohexadiene) decomposition (Taylor *et al.*, 1973; Taylor *et al.*, 1975). Reaction can be easily monitored by the change in UV absorbance at 478 nm. The dependence of the reaction rate on the substrate concentration demonstrated a saturation curve, which is typical for enzymatic reactions ($K_m = 9$ μM, $k_{cat} = 0.66\ s^{-1}$). The rate constant for degradation of the cyclohexadiene derivative at pH 7.5 was $0.26\ s^{-1}$, whereas the rate of uncatalyzed degradation was 7000 times lower ($k = 3.7 \times 10^{-5}\ s^{-1}$).

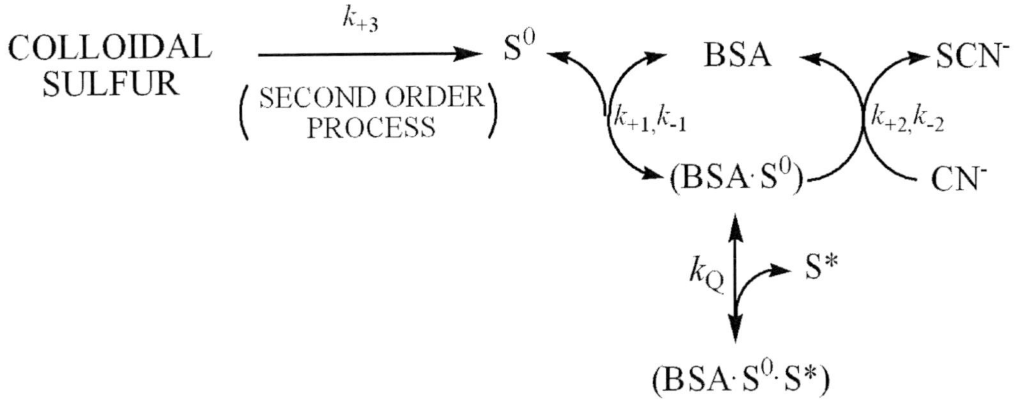

$$\frac{1}{v_{ss}} = \left[\frac{1}{k_{+1}[S]} + \frac{1+K_Q[S]}{k_{+2}[KCN]} + \frac{k_{-1}}{k_{+1}k_{+2}[S][KCN]}\right]\frac{1}{[BSA]} + \frac{1}{k_{+3}[S]^2}$$

Scheme 20.

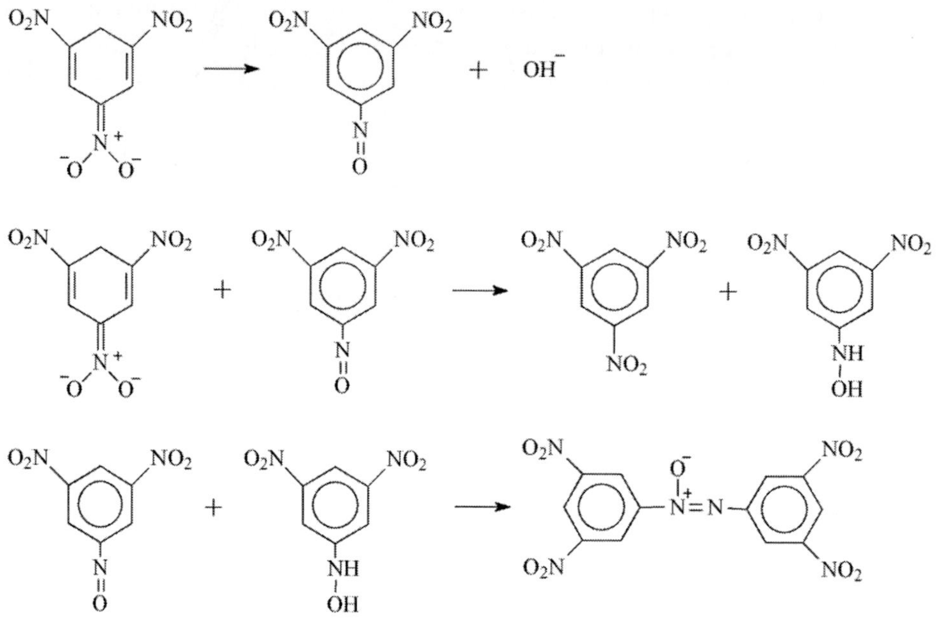

Scheme 21.

It was shown that a native structure of albumin was essential for the reaction. No activity was observed at pH 11-12 (conformational transition), in 8 M urea or SDS. According to ^{1}H NMR, UV-Vis spectrophotometry and mass spectrometry, the conversion of trinitrocyclohexadiene to 3,5,3',5''-tetranitroazoxibenzene proceeds via formation of trinitrobenzene (Scheme 21) (Taylor and Vatz, 1973).

The pH profile for the reaction allowed the authors (Taylor *et al.*, 1975) to suggest that the catalysis is provided by one deprotonated lysine residue with a pK_a of 8.4. It was shown that HSA lacking Lys-220, which was found to be the site of albumin's modification by fluoresceine isothiocyanate (Taylor *et al.*, 1976) and the residue involved in pyridoxal binding, is inert to Meisenheimer complex.

Taylor and co-authors (Taylor *et al.*, 1975) have proposed that the withdrawal of the proton from *ortho* position of trinitrociclodiene ring by the deprotonated lysine residue is a rate determining step of the reaction. This process is followed by the proton transfer from the protonated Lys residue to the nitro group. Subsequent OH group elimination leads to 3,5-dinitrobenzene. In this case, a water molecule rather hydroxyl ion is a leaving group. The formed nitroso compound interacts with the initial cyclodiene derivative to yield both 3,5-dinitrobenzene and dinitrophenylhydroxylamine. It is known (Popova *et al.*, 2010) that *N*-substituted hydroxylamines are reactive towards nitroso compounds with azoxy compounds being the products of condensation. Indeed, 3,3',5,5'-tetranitroazoxybenzene was found to be a final product of trinitrocyclohexadiene degradation in the presence of albumin (Taylor *et al.*, 1975).

3. Possible Applications of Serum Albumin's Catalytic Activities

The wide range of reactions catalyzed by serum albumin, together with its natural abundance and relatively high catalytic efficiency at extreme temperatures, make albumin an appealing candidate for biocatalytic applications, including bioprocesses in non-aqueous solvents. For example, Liu and Lemma-Gray utilized BSA to catalyze the isomerization of 1,2-benzisoxazole in pure acetonitrile (Liu and Lemma-Gray, 2001). BSA is an effective catalyst for the deprotonation of benzisoxazoles (Kikuchi *et al.*, 1996). In aqueous solution, BSA was found to catalyze the conversion of 5-nitrobenzoxazole into the correspondent salicylonitrile (Scheme 22) (Kikuchi *et al.*, 1996).

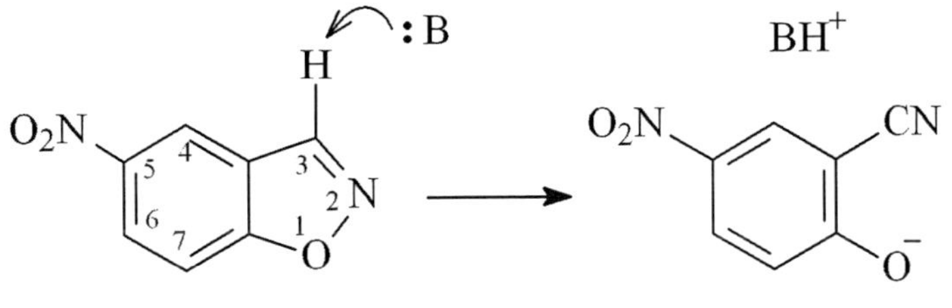

Scheme 22.

The catalysis showed a Michaelis-Menten behavior with an estimated $k_{cat} = 0.017 \pm 0.001\ s^{-1}$, $K_m = 720 \pm 68\ \mu M$ (Kikuchi *et al.*, 1996). The activity of BSA in acetonitrile was approximately 20% of that in water under similar conditions (Liu and Lemma-Gray, 2001). In acetonitrile, a Michaelis-Menten behavior was also exhibited, and an estimated catalytic efficiency (k_{cat}/K_M) of 8.77 $M^{-1}s^{-1}$ was achieved. Inhibition studies show that the active site may be the same as that responsible for pyridoxal binding (involving Lys-220). To explain the strong inhibitory effect of the reaction product on the reaction, the authors (Kikuchi *et al.*, 1996) also suggested that the product phenolate is stabilized by a cluster of positively charged arginine residues.

Another possible application of catalytic properties of serum albumin is the detoxification of harmful compounds at low substrate concentrations. One of the examples of this application was demonstrated by *Sogorb et al.*, who exploited the ability of rabbit serum albumin to hydrolyze carbamate carbaryl, eliminating the toxicity of this pesticide (Sogorb *et al.*, 2002).

Recombinant technology allows engineering and production of proteins with the desirable properties. The recombinant technology has been employed for HSA production as well. The success in this field has contributed to a wider application of HSA as a drug carrier in the clinical setting (Otagiri and Chuang, 2009). Scaled-up production of recombinant albumin (rHSA) in *Pichia pastoris* has made the protein to be used for pharmaceutical purposes (Kobayashi, 2006). This product exhibits good pharmacokinetics and biodistribution (Matsushita *et al.*, 2006). Thus, rHSA seems to be an ideal candidate for protein engineering. Increasing the bimolecular rate constant of albumin for organophosphates is a protein engineering challenge that could lead to a new class of bio-scavengers to be used against poisoning by nerve agents. Soman-albumin adducts detected by mass spectrometry can be useful for the diagnosis of soman exposure (Li *et al.*, 2008).

Domain I of HSA has great potential for further development as a "stand-alone" protein for its potential use as a drug delivery protein carrier due to its antioxidative activity and enolase-like activity (Matsushita *et al.*, 2004). In addition, the presence of a free cysteine residue allows relatively easy conjugation of the protein with a drug containing a free thiol moiety.

The esterase-like properties of HSA can be of practical use. Thus, a series of synthetic chromogenic and fluorogenic substrates for monitoring the arylesterase-like activity of albumins from various sources has been studied (Wolfbeis and Gürakar, 1987). The acetate, butyrate, caprylate, laurate, and palmitate esters of a coumarin dye were found to be efficiently hydrolyzed within the pH range 8.8-9.8, with the non-enzymatic rate being the highest for acetate and the lowest for laurate. A considerable increase in the hydrolytic activity was observed upon the addition of detergents, but not of Ca^{2+} and Mg^{2+} ions. The addition of one equivalent of lauric acid to BSA resulted in a 30% decrease in its activity. The results were interpreted in terms of the well-known affinity of albumins for long chain fatty acids. The observed catalytic activity of albumin provided the basis for a sensitive kinetic method for albumin quantitation. The method utilizes the protein's hydrolytic activity toward 7-lauroyl-3-(5-methyl-7-sulfonato-2-benzoxazolyl)-coumarin as a substrate; this particular substrate is suitable for both photometric and fluorometric assays (Gürakar and Wolfbeis, 1988).

If we consider the high albumin's concentration in human plasma (~0.6 mM), the esterase-like activity of HSA should also be taken into account in drug development. On the one hand, albumin can bind and hydrolyze ester bonds of a number of active drugs, thus decreasing their pharmacological effect. On the other hand, the esterase-like activity of HSA could be also used to convert an acetylated pro-drug into a functional drug, as can be illustrated by olmesartan medoxomil. For example, the crystallographic structure of the complex of HSA with a non-steroidal anti-inflammatory drugdiflunisal shows that one diflunisal molecule is bound to HSA in domain IIA, where it interacts with Tyr-150 (2.19 Å) and His-242 (3.46 Å) of HSA (Ghuman *et al.*, 2005). By utilizing acetylated diflunisal as a pro-drug, it might be possible to activate this drug through HSA's esterase activity, alter its binding orientation, and thus reduce its affinity to HSA.

Finally, Córdova *et al.* reported that BSA can catalyze ester hydrolysis at high temperatures (as high as 160 °C), which is well beyond the temperature limits reported for the enzymatic catalysis, including for enzymes from known hyperthermophiles (Córdova *et al.*, 2008). Furthermore, BSA exhibited a ~133-fold increase in its turnover number (k_{cat}) toward *p*-nitrophenyl palmitate upon the temperature increase from 70 to 150 °C. This data can serve to support the evolutionary hypothesis that promiscuous enzymes may have maximized the catalytic versatility of ancestral cells with small gene contents and limited enzyme resources. The authors (Córdova *et al.*, 2008) have suggested that promiscuous activity of albumins and their apparent origin from a common ancestor support the hypothesis that ancestral albumins may have performed catalytic functions in primitive life forms at high temperatures. Hyperthermophilic organisms, in their possible role as the earliest ancestors of life (Schwartzman and Lineweaver, 2004), would certainly have benefited from the synergy of promiscuity and catalysis at high temperatures. The combination of these two properties may have been necessary to meet the biochemical and survival requirements of hyperthermophilic ancestral cells. Though the key role of albumin-like proteins in high-temperature survival and adaptation is still a hypothesis, their functional versatility and resistance to harsh conditions allows one to speculate about albumins as a possible model for the early-stage development of primordial enzymes.

ACKNOWLEDGMENTS

We wish to thank the Russian Foundation for Basic Research (RFBR 09-04-01483), the RF President grant (NS-3185.2010.4), and the Siberian Branch of the Russian Academy of Sciences (the Integration grant #88) for financial support.

In: Serum Albumin: Structure, Functions and Health Impact ISBN: 978-1-62100-231-4
Editors: R. J. Alekseev and A. L. Rebane

Chapter 2

INTERACTION OF SERUM ALBUMIN WITH ANESTHETICS

Makoto Nishimoto,[1] Michio Yamanaka[2] and Hitoshi Matsuki[1,*]
[1]Department of Life System, Institute of Technology and Science,
The University of Tokushima, Tokushima, Japan
[2]Department of Chemistry, Faculty of Sciences, Kyushu University,
Higashi-ku, Fukuoka, Japan

ABSTRACT

The molecular mechanism of anesthesia is one of the long-standing unresolved problems in medical science. Although two representative theories of anesthesia, a protein receptor theory based on the direct binding of anesthetics to several signal receptor proteins in nerve membranes and a lipid membrane theory based on the indirect binding of anesthetics to nerve membranes with high content of lipids, have been argued up to now, the action mechanism has not yet been clarified. More recently, the emphasis has shifted from theories oflipid perturbation to the idea that anesthetics bind directly to specific proteins.Serum albumin is an abundant plasma protein transporting a wide variety of drugs and endogenous compounds and has been widely used for life-science studies. A number of studies on the binding of such drugs and compounds to serum albumin have been reported since pioneer works by Foster et al. in late 1950s. In the beginning of 1990s, Carter et al. determined the detailed molecular structure of serum albumin from the X-ray structural analysis, and subsequently the binding sites of several small ligands for serum albumin were identified on the structure. In such circumstances, serum albumin has been regarded a good model for anesthetic action, and the binding data of anesthetics to serum albumin examined by various physicochemical methods have been accumulated for the last several decades. Most of the binding studies of anesthetics to serum albumin showed that there exist weak but specific interactions between serum albumin and anesthetics, and crystallographic data suggested that all anesthetics bind fatty-acid binding sites on serum albumin without binding the unique site to each anesthetic. On the other hand, a comparative study of ligand interactions indicated that the binding mode of anesthetics is pronouncedly different from that of specific binders

[*]E-mail address: matsuki@bio.tokushima-u.ac.jp

such as fatty acids. Here model studies of anesthetic action by using serum albumin are reviewed, and characteristic binding modes of anesthetics to serum albumin are elucidated in connection with the anesthetic mechanism.

INTRODUCTION

Organic compounds with a small and simple structure are well known to induce anesthetic action more than a hundred years ago. However, it has not yet been clarified why such compounds show the action and which biomolecules they act on. Anesthetics and the anesthetic action have common features as follows. (1) No specificity of molecularstructure: various kinds of organic compounds such as ethers, alcohols and even inactive gases have anesthetic potency, indicating undoubtedly that functional groups needed for the anesthetic action cannot be identified. Figure 1 shows various molecular structures of anesthetics referred in this chapter. (2) High effective concentration: the EC_{50} (the concentration needed for 50% drug action) values of anesthetics are more than 1000 times larger than those of receptor-binding drugs. (3) Pressure reversal of anesthesia: pressure antagonisms the anesthetic action. (4) Cut off phenomenon: long-chain organic compounds do not possess the anesthetic potency. These characteristics of anesthetics distinctly describe that the action of anesthetic is remarkably different from that of most drugs biochemically or physiologically oriented.

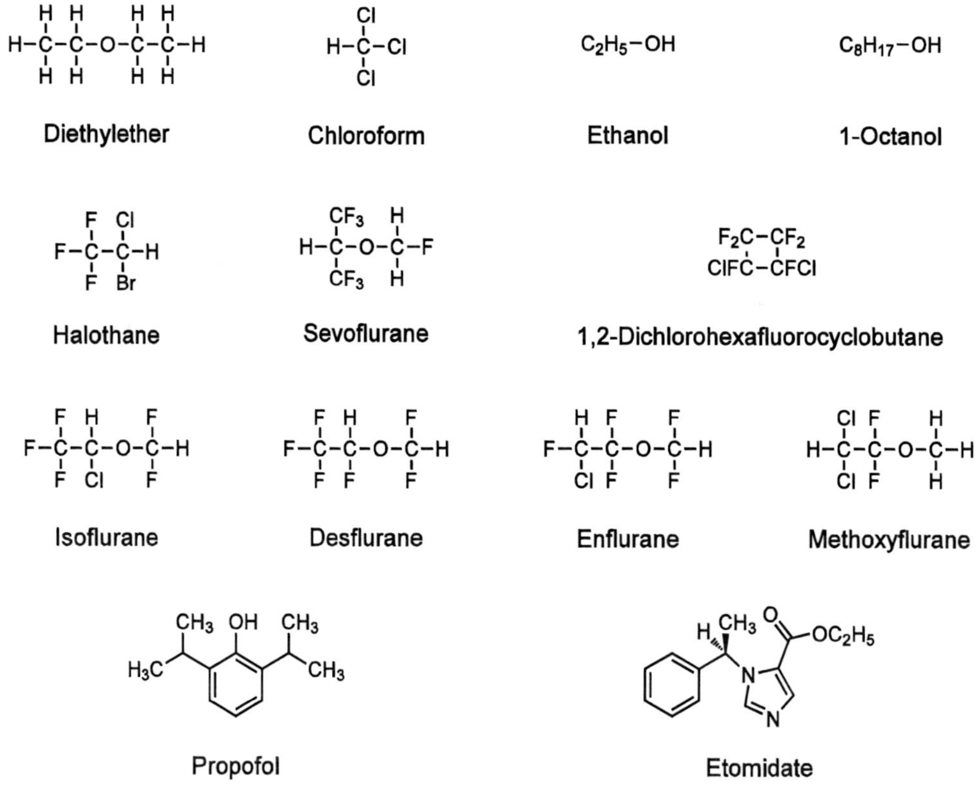

Figure 1. Molecular structures of inhalation anesthetics described in this chapter.

Meyer-Overton rule early in twentieth century showed well correlation between anesthetic potency and hydrophobicity of the anesthetic molecule and suggested that environments on which anesthetics act are lipophilic. Since then, anesthetics are commonly regarded as membrane-targeting drugs. Since biological membranes are composed of lipid bilayers and many proteins buried in the membrane, anesthetic research for both biomolecules has been done until now. Studies of the anesthetic effect on lipid bilayers have been flourished up to the middle of 1980s. This is called a lipid membrane theory, which insists that nonspecific binding of the anesthetic molecules to nerve membranes with high content of lipids changes the membrane properties as fluidity and phase state, and then the secondary effect on the membrane proteins causes anesthesia [1,2]. But, several objections to the lipid membrane theory together with the violation of the Meyer-Overton rule, namely low-temperature enhancement of anesthesia, effects of stereoisomers and nonimmobilizers, and cut off phenomenon, were proposed and it gradually lost the support of anesthetic researchers. During the backlash of the lipid membrane theory, a protein receptor theory [3-5], which explains that anesthesia is caused by the specific binding of anesthetic molecules to several signal receptor proteins in the membrane, became predominant and so popular in 1990s. Recent anesthetic studies concentrate on examinations of specific interactions between anesthetics and various kinds of proteins, and most researchers continue to look for the anesthetic binding sites in these proteins. In the background of a recent fashion of the protein receptor theory, a lot of anesthetic studies using aqueous globular proteins have been performed. Especially, one of the representative proteins, serum albumin, has been frequently used in model studies of anesthetic action.

Serum albumin is a protein contained greatly in blood plasma, occurring there at a concentration of about 0.6 mM and comprising 50-60% of the total plasma protein. The important roll of serum albumin is a vehicle to transport several endogenous compounds such as fatty acids, bilirubin, hemin, tryptophan, and so forth. These compounds bind serum albumin with high affinity. Serum albumin has been widely used in various life-science studies as a model protein because the high-purity reagent is abundantly available in low price. Hence, the physicochemical properties of serum albumin have been investigated in detail, and it turned out that serum albumin is a markedly unique protein. As one example, it is well known that serum albumintakes place structural changes depending on the solution pH. Aoki and Foster clarified from a method of electrophoresis in the 1960s [6,7] that bovine serum albumin (BSA) has different forms at various pHs, which are classified into expanded (E) and fast (F) forms in the acidic pH region, a normal (N) form in the neutral pH region, and a basic (B) form in the alkaline pH region. The physical quantities of BSA definitely change between two forms at certain pHs, which is called the structural transition of serum albumin. Other biochemical and biophysical properties are well served by comprehensive reviews [7-9]. In 1992, He and Carter [10] determined the high-resolution crystal structure of human serum albumin (HSA), also followed soon after by the structure of horse serum albumin [11]. This introduced structural information to studies of serum albumin, and these structures provided new insights into the binding sites of a lot of drugs including anesthetics.

In this chapter, we review the anesthetic studies performed on serum albumin until now. At first, the binding studies of anesthetics to serum albumin in the early stage are shown, and subsequently the studies from the viewpoint of the protein receptor theory performed in mainly 1990s are demonstrated. Next, the binding sites of anesthetics on

HSA identified by using the X-ray structural analysis and the specific interaction between HSA and anesthetics are explained. Finally, recent our idea for the intrinsic interaction mode of serum albumin with anesthetics is described.

1. Model Studies Based on Nonspecific Interactions

There were a few reports of the effect of inhalation anesthetics such as halothane and chloroform on serum albumin at an early stage [12-15], where partitioning studies from the solubility of these anesthetic gases were made, and the reports demonstrated that such anesthetics partition extensively into serum albumin. The interaction between serum albumin and anesthetics was first examined from the viewpoint of nonspecific interaction between them in the period of the lipid membrane theory.

1.1. Spectrophotometry

A research of anesthetic-serum albumin interaction in relation to the anesthetic mechanism was first reported by Mashimo and Ueda in 1982 [16]. They used a pH-sensitive dye, bromothymol blue (BTB), which is a negatively charged ligand and can bind the albumin molecule, and observed the color-change of BTB by binding of BTB to a BSA molecule. The binding inhibition by an inhalation anesthetic methoxyflurane was analyzed by a statistical mechanical theory derived. They showed that the Scatchard plot is inapplicable to the analysis of the binding parameters in the presence of low concentrations of anesthetics. But at the high concentrations, the binding constant and the binding number could be estimated because the binding parameter approaches a limiting value. It was revealed that methoxyflurane decreases the binding constant of BTB without changing the binding number. A few years later, they examined the change in surface potential of a BSA molecule due to the binding of BTB by combing the observation of the color-change with pH measurements of the bulk solution [17]. The surface potential of BTB binding site was estimated from the mismatch between the bulk pH and the color of the bound BTB. From the pH-color mismatch in the presence of anesthetics at high ionic strength, it was found that the mismatch is mainly caused by the anesthetic effect on the electrostatic potential of BSA surface interacting with BTB, not nonelectrostatic contribution at the binding region. Anesthetics such as diethyether, enflurane, and methoxyflurane decreased the surface potential, and the decrease was in excellent agreement with the clinical potencies of the anesthetics. Because a decrease in the surface potential by anesthetics would decrease the electrostatic force imposed on the water dipole and decompose the electrostricted water structure clustered around the surface charge, they described that the release of electrostricted water molecules increases the total volume. The hydration of BSA was investigated from a method of dielectric dispersion by Yoshida et al. [18] in later years. They indicated that halothane decreases the number of the strongly bound water molecules, whereas increases that of weakly bound water molecules, and the change is attributable to the change of bulk ion concentrations due to the binding of halothane to BSA.

1.2. Densitometry

An anesthetic effect on volumes of biomolecules is important to clarify the anesthetic mechanism because the volumes are related to the phenomenon of pressure reversal of anesthesia. Ueda and Mashimo [19] have also examined the volume behavior of BSA in the presence of an anesthetic diethylether by means of a high-precision oscillation densimeter. They clarified from the difference between the partial molar volumes of BSA at infinite dilution and the molar volume of dry BSA that the number of electrostricted water molecules at the surface of BSA in aqueous solutions at 20°C is estimated to be about 720. Figure 2(a) shows the apparent molar volumes of BSA in the solution as a function of diethylether concentration. Addition of diethylether to the BSA solution increased the apparent molar volume of BSA dose-dependently. They showed that 57.9 mmolal diethylether expands the partial molar volumes of BSA at 20°C by 0.59% and about 110 water molecules in about 720 electrostricted water molecules under the experimental condition are released from the BSA surface assuming that the expansion is caused mainly by melting of electrostricted water molecules.

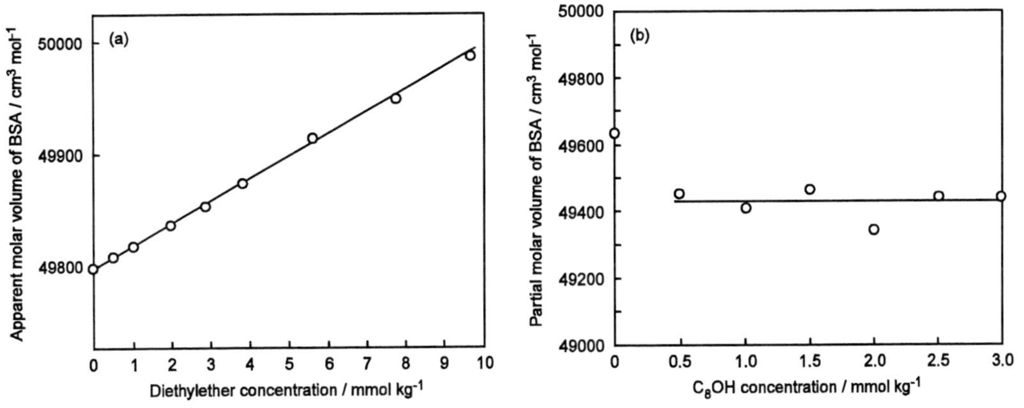

Figure 2. (a) Apparent molar volume of BSA versus diethylether concentration curve at 20°C. (b) Partial molar volume of BSA at infinite dilution versus C_8OH concentration curve at 25°C.

Yamanaka et al. [20] have also investigated the volume behavior of BSA in the absence and presence of medium chain alcohol octanol (C_8OH). They measured the densities of BSA solutions as a function of BSA and C_8OH concentrations at 25°C and analyzed the density data by use of thermodynamic equations describing the volume behavior of protein-ligand mixtures. The partial molar volumes of BSA at infinite dilution are plotted against C_8OH concentration in Figure 2(b). It was seen that the partial molar volumes in the presence of C_8OH are small as compared with that in the absence of C_8OH. By using the concentration dependence of the partial molar volumes of BSA and C_8OH at infinite dilution with a Langmuir-type binding isotherm, they calculated the volume change of BSA-C_8OH binding. The resulting volume-change value was large negative (-109 cm^3 mol^{-1}), that is, C_8OH reduces the BSA volume. They explained that the shrinkage of BSA volume by C_8OH may be caused by the nonspecific solvent effect and the hydrophobic interaction between C_8OH molecules at their binding sites on BSA. Since the positive volume change is required for the pressure reversal of anesthesia,they also concluded that this BSA-C_8OH system does not undergo the pressure-anesthetic antagonism and BSA may not be a relevant proteinto the anesthetic mechanism. The obtained result for the BSA-C_8OH system was inconsistent with that for the above-mentioned BSA-diethylether system: diethylether expands the BSA volume while C_8OH conversely reduces the volume. This peculiar volume behavior of BSA is hardly observable for any other globular proteins and seems to be closely related to the difference in ligand sensibility of BSA to anesthetics with different hydrophobicity, which will be discussed later.

2. Model Studies Based on Specific Interactions

Franks and Lieb [3-5] have demonstrated that the Meyer-Overton rule can be reproduced using a soluble protein like a firefly luciferase. The protein is inactivated by clinical doses of an inhalation anesthetic in the total absence of lipid. And then, a number of model studies directing toward specific interactions between a protein and anesthetics have been performed. Such studies for serum albumin were undertaken early in 1990s,and subsequently, Eckenhoff's group energeticallystudied the specific interaction between serum albumin and inhalation anesthetics, especially, halothane (Refer to their review [21]). Here we primarily review their results obtained for the specific interaction.

2.1. ^{19}F Nuclear Magnetic Resonance

The specific interaction of serum albumin with anesthetics has been first reported by Dubois and Evers [22]. They examined the binding of one of fluorinated inhalation anesthetics, isoflurane, to BSA by using transverse relaxation time (T_2) of ^{19}F Nuclear Magnetic Resonance (^{19}F-NMR). The T_2 value of the trifluoromethyl group of isoflurane in the BSA solutions increased with isoflurane concentration but the values in the lysozyme and poly(L-lysine) had no concentration dependence (see Figure 3(a)). They indicated that the binding is saturable and determined the value of the dissociation constant (K_D) as 1.4 mM. The binding was eliminated either by coincubation with oleic acid (6 mol/mol of BSA) or by conversion of BSA to its expanded form by titration to pH 2.5. Further, this study was extended to other fluorinated anesthetics [23], halothane, methoxyflurane, and sevoflurane, and the K_D values were determined for the anesthetics (halothane, 1.3 mM; methoxyflurane, 2.6 mM; sevoflurane, 4.5 mM), respectively. The three anesthetics all inhibited isoflurane binding to BSA in a competitive manner with a similar inhibition constant (K_I: halothane, 1.3 mM; methoxyflurane, 2.5 mM; sevoflurane, 5.4 mM) to each anesthetic's K_D, and the fatty acid-binding domains in BSA were identified as probable sites of these volatile anesthetics. Similar T_2 measurements of ^{19}F-NMR have been also done by Xu et al. [24] to investigate stereoselective binding of isoflurane to BSA. Although the S(+) and R(–) enantiomers, and the racemic mixture exhibited no stereoselectivity in K_D values (1.3 ± 0.2 mM), they observed the stereoselectivity in dynamic binding parameters, that is, the S(+) enantiomer binds BSA with slower association and dissociation rates than the R(–) one. Because the dissociation rate constant measures the strength of the binding, they concluded that the S(+) enantiomer is more potent than the R(–) one.

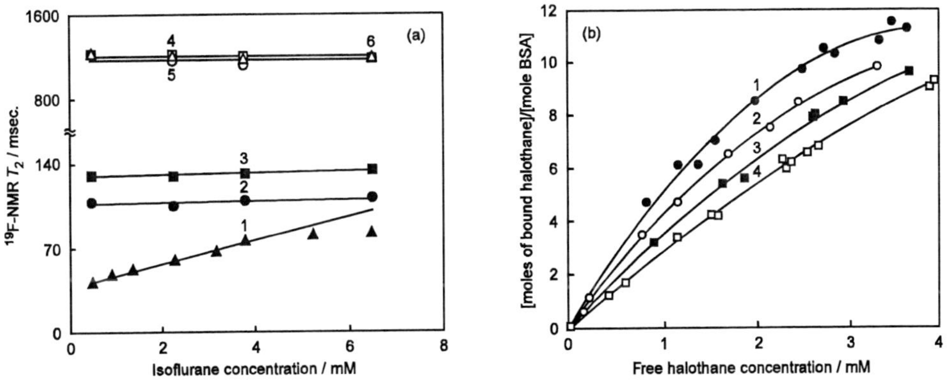

Figure 3. (a) Transverse relaxation time of isoflurane trifluoromethyl group versus isoflurane concentration at 22°C: (1) BSA (6 mg ml^{-1}), (2) BSA in the presence of oleic acid (6:1 oleic acid/BSA molar ratio, (3) BSA at pH 2.5, (4) lysozyme (6 mg ml^{-1}), (5) poly(L-lysine) (6 mg ml^{-1}), (6) buffer alone. (b) Binding isotherms of halothane to BSA constructed from ^{19}F-NMR measurements. Bound halothane expressed by molar ratio of bound halothane to BSA is plotted against free halothane concentration: (1) 10°C, (2) 22°C, (3) 30C, (4) 37°C.

Yoshida et al. have designed a novel NMR tube [25], which can obtain anesthetic signals from gas and water phases simultaneously while maintaining the equilibrium condition. They measured the ^{19}F-NMR spectra of the BSA solution in the presence of halothane with the novel tube and determined the bound and free halothane concentrations in water by comparing the NMR signal strengths in the absence and presence of BSA. The resulting binding isotherms of halothane to BSA are shown in Figure 3(b). It is seen that the halothane binding to BSA is saturable. Assuming the Langmuir type interaction, the values of K_D and maximum binding number (B_{max}) were calculated to be 2.6 mM, 19.3 at 10°C and 10.9 mM, 34.5 at 37°C, respectively. The values of enthalpy (ΔH) and entropy (ΔS) associated with the transfer of an anesthetic from water to BSA, which were evaluated from the K_D values and the temperature dependence of K_D, were both negative.Although the general consensus of hydrophobic interaction is entropy-driven (classical hydrophobic effect [26]), the binding of halothane to BSA was enthalpy-driven (nonclassical hydrophobic effect [27]), compensating the opposing effect of ΔS with negative ΔH. They pointed out that BSA is a specific protein and the negative ΔS may be attributable to the conformational change of BSA due to the halothane binding. Recently Shikii et al. [28] have examined the interaction of halothane and HSA by using of one dimensional and two-dimensional ^{1}H-^{19}F-NMR techniques including measurements of diffusion coefficients of halothane. As they observed the strong intermolecular nuclear Overhauser effects on HSA and halothane complex and clear decreases in diffusion coefficients of halothane in the presence of HSA, they concluded that there is the distinct interaction of HSA with halothane.

2.2. Photoaffinity Labeling

Eckenhoff et al. [29] have developed a novel direct photoaffinity labeling method in order to determine the binding characteristics of halothane to serum albumin. They used a radioactive ^{14}C-halothane in the binding study. Exposure of ^{14}C-halothane to UV light causes photolysis, with the products of ^{14}C labeled chlorotrifluoroethyl and Br radicals [30], then the ethyl radical is expected to covalently bind rapidly and irreversibly to certain sites of a protein in close proximity to the reversible pharmacologic binding sites. They applied this technique to BSA and quantitated the covalently bound ^{14}C-halothane to BSA by scintillation counting after precipitation, filtration, and washing of BSA-labeled halothane complex. In the photoaffinity labeling method, the native structure of a protein is lost, but it has several merits that it separates specific from nonspecific binding, requires far less protein than ^{19}F-NMR and chromatographic methods, and does not require a reporter group such as an aromatic residue and spin label in the vicinity of the anesthetic binding site.

Figure 4(a) illustrates the ^{14}C-halothane binding to BSA as a function of halothane concentration at a room temperature (ca. 22°C). Since the total binding isotherm obtained from the binding experiments consists of specific and nonspecific labeling of ^{14}C-halothane, the contribution of the nonspecific labeling was estimated at pH 2 (an expanded form of BSA) and subtracted from the total binding isotherm. A specific binding isotherm with clear evidence of saturation was obtained together with a smaller $K_D$value between 0.3 and 0.5 mM than those determined by other methods. They explained that the photolabeling K_D values are indeed an underestimation of true equilibrium values because of irreversible depletion of the sites at high anesthetic concentrations. By competitive binding experiments with other kinds of anesthetics, all anesthetics inhibited photochemical incorporation of label in a dose-dependent manner (K_I: unlabeled halothane, 0.36 mM; chloroform, 1.26 mM; methoxyflurane, 2.66 mM, isoflurane, 1.47 mM; diethylether, 45.5 mM; ethanol, 1040 mM). One example of the competitive experiments for unlabeled halothane is shown in Figure 4(b). Oleate and BSA conformational change induced by low pH or adding guanidine hydrochloride also inhibited the label incorporation. They reported later that the halothane binding to BSA investigated by this technique is much more different from that of another globular proteins, myoglobin (Mgb) [31].

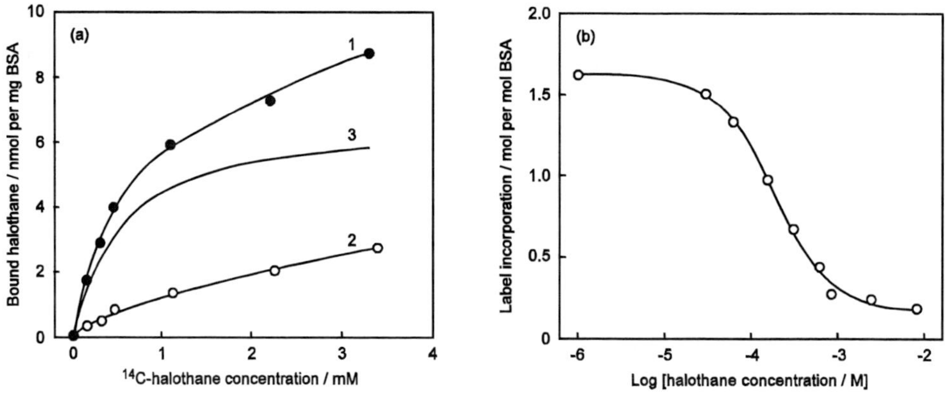

Figure 4. (a) Binding isotherms of halothane to BSA constructed from photoaffinity labeling measurements at 25°C: (1) total label incorporation at pH 7.0, (2) nonspecific labeling (total labeling at pH 2.0, (3) specific labeling obtained from the difference between total and specific labeling. (b) Competition curve for ^{14}C-halothane (0.1 mM) labeling of BSA using unlabeled halothane as a competitor at 22°C.

Recently, Bright et al. [32] have synthesized a novel analog of an intravenous anesthetic etomidate in which the ethoxy group has been replaced by an azide group, and which can be used as a photolabel to identify etomidate-binding sites. The azide group produces a highly reactive nitrene on illumination and has been used as the photoactivatable group. After they confirmed that the acyl azide analog exhibits almost the same anesthetic action as etomidate, they used the analog as a photolabeling reagent to identify etomidate binding sites to HSA. Two anesthetic binding sites on HSA were identified by using HPLC coupled with a mass spectrometry. One site is a well-characterized drug-binding site I located in subdomain IIA in HSA, and the second site is a binding site of another intravenous anesthetic propofol located in subdomain IIB, both of which sites are described in the latter section of structural analysis for HSA.

2.3. Fluorometry

Fluorescence measurements are frequently employed for experiments of protein-ligand binding. Johansson et al. [33,34] have observed the binding of inhalation anesthetics, halothane and chloroform, to BSA and HSA by monitoring intrinsic tryptophan fluorescence quenching. There are two tryptophans in BSA, at positions 134 (subdomain IB) and 212 (subdomain IIA), where the tryptophan at position 134 is thought to be more exposed to the aqueous solvent compared with that at position 212. HSA has a single tryptophan at position 214. Since if anesthetics with heavy atoms (Cl or Br) like halothane and chloroform bind in close proximity to the tryptophan residue in serum albumin, the intrinsic fluorescence of the tryptophan residue is quenched, hence, the binding around the residue can be detected. Advantages of this method are that it is more sensitive and nondestructive compared with the photoaffinity labeling technique, however, the method is limited to detect anesthetic binding to proteins at sites containing aromatic residues such as phenylalanine, tyrosine, and tryptophan.

The fluorescence quenching of tryptophan residues in BSA by halothane at 25°C is demonstrated in Figure 5(a). Halothane quenched the tryptophan fluorescence of BSA in a dose-dependent, saturable manner with a K_D of 1.8 ± 0.2 mM and a Hill number of 1.0 ± 0.1 (curve 1). The quenching ability of halothane was markedly reduced at pH 3.0 (full uncoiling of BSA) with loss of saturable binding (curve 2). The effect of halothane on L-tryptophan and apomyoglobin which has two tryptophan residues at positions 7 and 14 was much smaller than that on BSA (curves 3 and 4). They also estimated the K_D value at position 134 by assuming that the halothane-binding site in the vicinity of position 212 in BSA is similar to that of position 214 in HSA (K_D = 3.9 mM). The resulting value was 1.3 mM, indicating that the affinity of binding site including the position 134 is stronger than that including the position 212. The results of circular dichroism spectroscopy exhibited that there is no measurable effect on the secondary structure of BSA by halothane binding. Furthermore, the analysis of Stern-Volmer plot and fluorescence lifetime revealed that the majority of the quenching is due to a static mechanism of anesthetic binding. Almost similar results were obtained for the effect of chloroform binding to BSA (K_D = 2.7 mM) and HSA (K_D = 5.6 mM) [34]. Therefore, they concluded that this study provides experimental support for the theory that structurally different inhalation anesthetics may occupy the same domains on protein targets.

Takehara et al. [35] have examined the binding characteristics of terminally substituted alkane analogs (C_nX: X = COOH, OH, CHO, NH_2, $CONH_2$) to BSA by a method of fluorescence titration. They performed a competitive binding assay using a fluorescent probe, 8-anilino-naphthalenesulfonate (ANS). ANS is one of specific binders to serum albumin (association constant (K_A): 1.42 × 10^6 M, B_{max}: 3.81 in BSA) and fluoresces strongly in hydrophobic environments but is almost nonfluorescent in water. Figure 5(b) shows the fluorescence inhibition of ANS bound to BSA by various kinds of decane analogs at 25°C. C_9COOH completely quenched the fluorescence of ANS bound to BSA, whereas $C_{10}OH$ and C_9CHO decreased the fluorescence intensity about 40% of the initial intensity. In contrast, $C_{10}NH_2$ and C_9CONH_2 decreased the fluorescence not more than 20% of the initial intensity. The inhibition of these ligands increased with an increase in hydrophobic chain length and there existed an inflection point on the site-occupancy curves of C_nCOOH with a longer chain. On the basis of these data, they classified the binding mode of C_nX to BSA into three types: two of them (Goup-I (anionic: C_nCOOH) and Group-II (nonionic: C_nOH and C_nCHO)) are detectable with the ANS fluorescence and the remaining one (Group-3 (cationic: C_nNH_2 and C_nCONH_2)) is not detectable with the fluorescence.

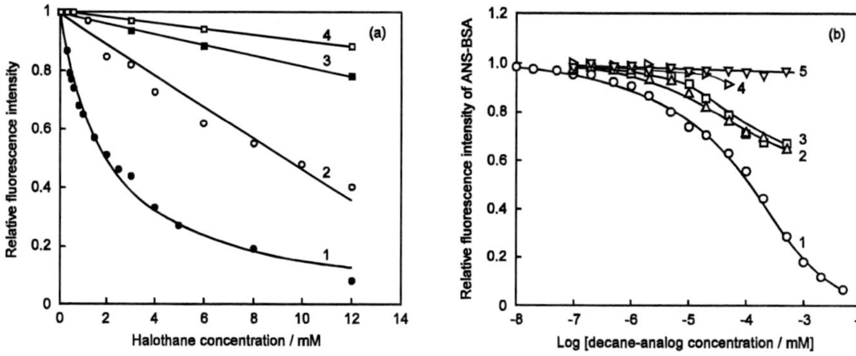

Figure 5. (a) Halothane quenching of tryptophan fluorescence in BSA at 25°C: (1) BSA of 5 μM at pH 7.0, (2) BSA of 5 μM at pH 3.0, (3) free tryptophan of 10 μM, (4) equine apomyoglobin of 5 μM at pH 7.0. (b) Decane analog quenching of ANS-BSA fluorescence at pH 7.4 and 25°C: (1) C_9COOH, (2) C_9CHO, (3) $C_{10}OH$, (4) C_9CONH_2, (5) $C_{10}NH_2$. The concentrations of ANS and BSA were 10.3 and 0.73 μM.

They also applied the similar treatment to HSA with another fluorescence measurement for an above-mentioned tryptophan residue in HSA [36]. In HSA, there are three florescence-active ANS binding sites including the tryptophan residue, and they are classified into two types by the affinity for ANS. It turned out that C_nCOOH binds to all three ANS binding sites with no fluorescence quenching of tryptophan, C_nCHO binds only to the site including the tryptophan residue, C_nOH binds to the site not including the residue, while C_nNH_2 does not bind to any of the three ANS binding sites. They explained that the different quenching behavior of the tryptophan fluorescence between C_nCHO and C_nOH is attributable to the difference in LUMO energy levels of these species.

2.4. Hydrogen Exchange

A hydrogen exchange method has been used by Eckenhoff et al. [31,37] to measure the effects of anesthetics and other perturbations such as temperature and pressure on a protein.

This assay is a method that exchanges hydrogens of amide bonds on peptide linkages in a protein for radioactive tritiums and detects the retained tritiums (bound to the protein) by scintillation counting in a similar manner as a photoaffinity labeling method. The hydrogen exchange technique is a very sensitive measure of shifts between folded and unfolded equilibrium, namely the ligand effect on the magnitude of the equilibrium constant. Specific binding to the native tertiary structure of a protein shifts the equilibrium toward more folded conformers, exposing internal amide hydrogens less often and thus slowing hydrogen exchange with water, whereas nonspecific binding shifts the equilibrium toward less folded conformers, resulting in more rapid exchange of the normally protected amide hydrogens with hydrogens of water. In other words, the slow hydrogen exchange corresponds to the stabilization of the protein while the rapid exchange does to the destabilization.

The hydrogen-tritium exchange-out curves for BSA in the absence and presence of halothane are drawn in Figure 6(a). Halothane decelerated the exchange rate of the amide hydrogens in a dose-dependent fashion, meaning stabilization of BSA by the preferential binding to the native, folded state. The protection factor ratio (PFR) was calculated by dividing the time required for a given hydrogen to exchange under the different conditions (with and without halothane), and then the change in Gibbs free energy of the fold state in the presence of halothane ($\Delta\Delta G$) was determined by use of the equation $\Delta\Delta G = -RT\ln$ (PFR). At 10 mM halothane, the values of PFR and $\Delta\Delta G$ were 27 and -2.04 kcal mol^{-1}. This fact implies that slowly exchanging BSA hydrogens are increased by up to 27-fold with 10 mM halothane and halothane brings about the stabilization of BSA as reflected by the negative $\Delta\Delta G$ values. This result of hydrogen exchange for BSA formed a striking contrast to that for Mgb [31]. The PFR values of Mgb were depressed by halothane and the $\Delta\Delta G$ values conversely had positive values, suggesting the destabilization of Mgb by binding of halothane to an intermediate or completely unfolded conformer. They concluded that halothane binds specifically with high (submillimolar) affinity to BSA, but either nonspecifically or with considerably lower affinity to Mgb.

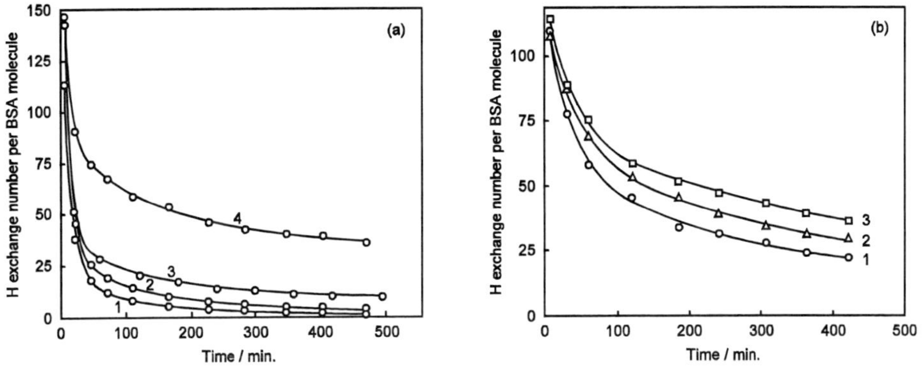

Figure 6. (a) Halothane effect on hydrogen-tritium exchange-out from BSA at pH 7.4, 1M guanidine HCl, and 37°C: (1) halothane concentration = 0 mM, (2) 1 mM, (3) 3 mM, (4) 10 mM. (b) Pressure effect on hydrogen-tritium exchange-out from BSA 37°C: (1) BSA at 1 atm, (2) BSA in the presence of 6 mM halothane at 200 atm, (3) BSA in the presence of 6 mM halothane at 1 atm.

Several factors affecting the hydrogen exchange for BSA in the presence of halothane were inquired [37]. The temperature dependence of the $\Delta\Delta G$ values was evaluated by comparing the values produced by 6 mM halothane at two temperatures. The obtained $\Delta\Delta G$ values were -1.53 kcal mol^{-1} at 22°C and -1.17 kcal mol^{-1} at 37°C, which gave the enthalpy ($\Delta\Delta H$) value of -8.3 kcal mol^{-1} at 22°C, meaning that the stabilization becomes stronger at a low temperature. The effect of pressure on the hydrogen exchange is shown in Figure 6(b). Although hydrostatic pressure of about 100 MPa uniformly caused the PFR values of pure BSA to decrease, pressure (200 MPa) partially reversed the stabilization produced by a relatively high concentration (6 mM) of halothane. On the other hand, these effects on the hydrogen exchange for Mgb were much smaller than those for BSA, the stereoselective effect of isoflurane was only slightly observed for BSA. Further, one of nonimmobilizers (anesthetic-like compounds that do not satisfy the Meyer-Overton correlation) 1,2-dichlorohexafluorocyclobutane destabilized both BSA and Mgb.

2.5. Calorimetry

Calorimetry is a powerful and informative technique for thermodynamic characterization of physical properties of biomolecules such as proteins and lipid membranes. Differential scanning calorimetry (DSC) can detect thermal structural transitions as a protein denaturation from the folded stated to the unfolded state while isothermal scanning calorimetry (ITC) can detect thermal energies of ligand binding to a protein directly.

The DSC study of the anesthetic action on a protein was first reported by Ueda et al. [38], which showed destabilization of firefly luciferase by ethanol. Subsequently, Tanner et al. [39,40] have studied the effect of halothane on the thermally induced unfolding transition of BSA by DSC. Figure 7(a) depicts the DSC thermograms of BSA solution in the absence and presence of halothane. The thermal denaturation temperature of BSA increased by adding halothane, and halothane stabilized the folded state of this protein, This result was well consistent with that obtained from the hydrogen exchange technique [31,37], and they explained that this thermal stabilization of BSA is caused by binding of halothane to the binding sites of native BSA specifically. From the thermodynamic consideration of a Gibbs energy of stabilization by halothane binding, the thermal stabilization of BSA was proved to be linked to the binding of about one halothane molecule at the lower concentrations and about six at the higher concentrations. They also studied the halothane effect on several kinds of globular proteins and reported that the thermal stabilization by halothane is brought about only in serum albumin [39] although the anesthetic sensibility of proteins markedly changes depending on the kinds of the protein.

Regarding the ITC studies on serum albumin-anesthetic interactions, first report was also done by Ueda and Yamanaka [41]. They did the direct binding study to estimate the ΔH value of anesthetic-protein complex formation by using ITC: the exact thermodynamic equations of ligand binding to a protein was derived and the averaged ΔH value of chloroform binding to BSA obtained by ITC was analyzed together with the equations. The averaged ΔH value was determined to be -10.37 kJ mol^{-1}, namely the chloroform binding was enhanced at a low temperature. The binding was saturable and characterized by the Langmuir adsorption isotherms. The Scatchard plots constructed by fitting free and bound chloroform concentrations were nonlinear, and then two binding modes (high- and low-affinity binding classes) were analyzed. Here the high-affinity interaction was estimated at the lowest choloroform/BSA concentration ratio, where almost all added chloroform molecules are bound to BSA, while the low-affinity interaction was estimated at the highest choloroform/BSA concentration ratio, where almost all added chloroform-binding sites on BSA are occupied. The K_D and B_{max} values were 0.47 mM and 3.7 for the high-affinity binding, and 5.29 mM and 13.2 for the low-affinity binding, respectively. They concluded with respect to the anesthetic-protein binding mode and the temperature dependence of anesthetic potency that the negative ΔH value of transfer of anesthetics from water to macromolecules (proteins and lipid membranes) is not limited to the selected signal proteins and the sign of the ΔH value is irreverent to the temperature dependence of anesthetic potency because the anesthetic potency is a function of the activity of anesthetic molecules, not the concentration.

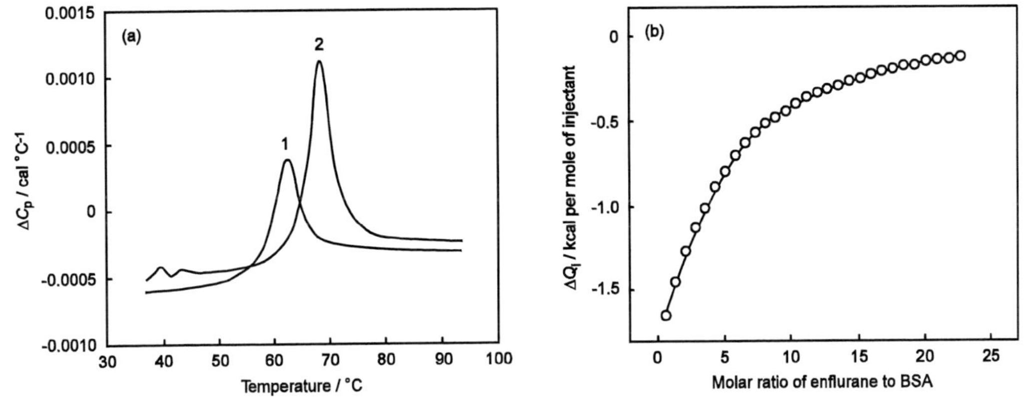

Figure 7. (a) DSC thermograms (differential heat capacity) of BSA (2 mg ml^{-1}) in the absence (1) and presence of 7 mM halothane (2) at pH 7.0. (b) Binding profile of enflurane to BSA measured by ITC at 20°C. 15 mMenflurane solution was titrated into 0.15 mM BSA solution and the change in the heat content of the solution for *i*th injection was plotted as a function of the molar ratio of enflurane to BSA.

Sawas et al. [42] have investigated the binding of four haloether anesthetics (desflurane, isoflurane, enflurane, and sevoflurane), a haloalkane anesthetic (halothane), and an intravenous anesthetic (propofol) to BSA and HSA from ITC in detail. The titration curve of enflurane solutions into a BSA solution is shown in Figure 7(b). The binding of all anesthetics to BSA and HSA was exothermic with the ΔH values between -3 and -6 kcal mol^{-1} for BSA, and the differences were largely ascribed to entropic contributions. Competition experiments suggested that all anesthetics share the same sites in albumin at low concentrations (B_{max} = 2 for propofol and 3 for the remaining anesthetics). The temperature dependence of the ΔH values yielded negative change in heat capacities (ΔC_p). From the comparison of the ΔC_p values with those calculated using the molecular modeling program for burial of each anesthetic in a hydrophobic pocket and the substitution experiments of heavy water for light water, they speculated that solvent restructuring, resulting from the release of water bound to anesthetic and anesthetic-binding sites, is a dominant and favorable contribution to the binding enthalpy and entropy.

Liu and Eckenhoff [43] have also studied anesthetic binding to HSA by ITC. They showed that the binding affinity of propofol to HSA has a K_D of 0.065 mM and a stoichiometry of ca. 2, whereas the binding affinity of halothane has a K_D of 1.6 mM and a stoichiometry of ca. 7. Anesthetic-HSAinteractions were exothermic, but propofol binding was enthalpy-driven process while halothane binding was entropy-driven process. Taking into account of molecular properties of propofol and halothane and ligand-protein contact, they explained thatthe stronger binding of propofol as compared with the less potent anesthetic halothane might be due to the combination of hydrogen bonding, stronger van der Waals and hydrophobic interactions at their two principal sites. They next examined the binding of other kinds of anesthetics, isoflurane and enflurane to HSA [44]. It was found that isoflurane binds to a single site of HSA with high affinity but smaller total enthalpy than enflurane that binds to two sites. Competitive experiments indicated that isoflurane and enflurane share one binding site, which also binds propofol. Another enflurane site binds propofol but not isoflurane. Taking into account the difference in dipole moment between isoflurane (2.0 debye) and enflurane (0.7 debye) and the salt concentration dependence of the binding, it turned out that one site is more polar and prefers isoflurane, and the other site is less polar and binds only enflurane. They suggested from the fact that weak polar interactions confer remarkable selectivity and differences in drug action.

2.6. Chromatography

Chan et al. [45] have introduced ananalyticalchromatography for the purpose of directly measuring ligand binding to a protein and applied this approach to the halothane binding to BSA and Mgb. They showed in zonal elution profiles from columns that the halothane binding to BSA is characterized as low affinity and multisite while to Mgb as strictly nonspecific. The immobilization of BSA in the column by low pH (3.0), denaturant (3M guanidine HCl), and specific binder (a saturating concentration of myristate) all decreased the halothane binding. They calculated from the values of apparent K_D and B_{max} from the continuous elution chromatography and obtained to be 1.3 mM and 2.1 for higher-affinity sites and 17.5 mM and 21.8 for lower-affinity ones, respectively.

Liu et al. [43] made a comparison of halothane and propofol binding to HSA by using this chromatographic technique. Figure 8(a) shows zonal elution profiles of HSA in the absence and presence of halothane or propofol. The zonal retention time of propofol was considerably large compared to that of halothane. The data of chromatography indicated clearly that the binding affinity of the propofol-HSA complex is much stronger than that of the halothane-HSA one, which were in good agreement with the ITC results mentioned in the previous section. The strong interaction between HSA and propofol was also proved from the continuous elution chromatography, which gave the apparent K_D value of 0.17 mM and the B_{max} value of 1.8.

2.7. Biochemical Assay

Eckenhoff's group has sought the location of anesthetic binding sites in serum albumin by combining biochemical assay such as enzyme digestion and site-directed mutagenesis with various physicochemical measurements described above. First, they did amino-acid resolution of halothane binding sites in serum albumin by proteolysis and microsequencing [46]. BSA and HSA photolabeled with ^{14}C-halothane was digested by cyanogen bromide and each fragment was separated by SDS-PAGE. The purified fragments containing significant labels were sequenced by a protein sequencer. It was found that BSA has a higher affinity for halothane than HSA and contained two specifically labeled sites. One was a diffuse labeling site from Trp-212 to Leu-217, the other was a discrete and higher affinity-labeling site between Trp-134 and Gly-135. On the other hand, HSA contained only a single labeled site. They suggested from the results that aromatic residues are important as a feature of binding sites of inhalation anesthetics.

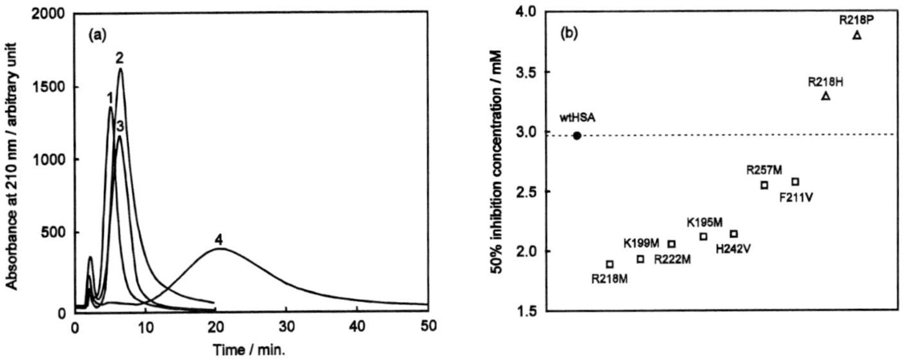

Figure 8. (a) Anesthetic binding to HSA measured by zonal elution chromatography at pH 7.0 and 25°C: (1) 10 mM halothane without HSA, (2) 0.5 mMpropofol without HSA, (3) 10 mM halothane with HSA, (4) 0.5 mMpropofol with HSA. (b) 50% inhibition concentration of specific site-directed mutants of HSA. The inhibition effect for each mutant was estimated from the quenching of tryptophan fluorescence of HSA.

They next examined another candidate for an anesthetic binding site [47], that is, a large hydrophobic cavity in domain III that contains Tyr-411 as a lining residue, by using a technique of site-directed mutagenesis with several physicochemical methods. Four kinds of HSA, recombinant wild type HSA (wtHSA), two single mutants (W214L and W214E), and one doublemutant (W214L/Y411W (dmHSA)) in which the tryptophan residue was transferred from 214 (interdomain cleft) position to 411 (domain III cavity) position, were used in this study.The photoaffinity labeling measurements showed that total label incorporation into the single mutants decreases, whereas the label into dmHSA increases due to the large increase in label in the 411 site. Halothane quenched the tryptophan fluorescence arising from Trp-214 (wtHSA) or Trp-411 (dmHSA). Isoflurane also quenched about half of the wtHSA fluorescence emission. In the presence of a 10-fold molar excess of myristate, the ability of halothane or isoflurane to quench Trp-411 was essentially eliminated by myristate in contrast to the Trp-214 position. In amide hydrogen-tritium exchange, the exchange rate of wtHSA was about 2-fold slower than BSA under the same conditions, indicating that wtHSA is more stable than BSA. All three mutants were less stable as compared with wtHSA, the stability decreased in the order of wtHSA> W214E > W214L >dmHSA. Halothane stabilized both wtHSA and three mutants, but there were some differences. Halothane stabilized W214E more than W214L. And the stabilization effect of isoflurane was weaker than that of halothane. The data suggested that the anesthetic binding in 214 interdomain cleft and 411 domain III cavity has similar character to each other, but there exists different selectivity for anesthetics. Further it was shown that myristate competes with anesthetic binding in the domain III cavity while allosterically enhances the binding in the interdomain cleft.

Site-directed mutants were also employed by Liu et al. [48] for an examination of the role of electrostatic interactions in HSA. They introduced site-directed mutagenesis in close proximity to Trp-214 in HSA and made nine kinds of HSA mutants. In the mutants, seven single mutants (K195M, K199M, R218M, R218P, R218H, R222M, and R257M) replaced positively charged residues with uncharged ones, one single mutant (H242V) replaced an uncharged polar residue with a uncharged nonpolar residue, and one single mutant (F211V) replaced an aromatic residue with an uncharged nonpolar residue. Structural geometry analysis of the HSA-halothane predicted an absence of significant electrostatic interactions. Physicochemical measurements (fluorometry, chromatography, and hydrogen exchange) were performed on these mutants. The IC_{50} (the concentration needed for 50% inhibition) values determined from fluorescence quenching of Trp-214 residue by halothane for seven mutants are illustrated together with that of wtHSA in Figure 8(b). The IC_{50} value of halothane for wtHSA was about 2.9 mM. The charged to uncharged mutations (K195M, K199M, R218M, R222M, and R257M) decreased the IC_{50} values by 10-35%, indicating environmental improvement in halothane binding in the Trp-214 binding site. H242V and F211V also decreased the IC_{50} values. Only R218P and R218H increased the IC_{50} values. The change in the IC_{50} values of halothane among the mutants well correlates with the change in the residue volume difference, which is obtained from the difference between the residue volume of wtHSA and that of a mutant. Since all mutations in this study shift to an increase in cavity volume, it was found that enlarging cavity due to smaller residue substitution tends to reduce halothane-binding affinity. The global protein stability evaluated from hydrogen exchange for the mutants almost exhibited stabilization of HSA. Furthermore, an increase in ionic strength also enhanced both regional (tryptophan region) and global halothane binding. They concluded from these facts that positive and negative electrostatic interactions either do not contribute or diminish halothane binding of HSA, suggesting that the binding of halothane is controlled primary by the more general hydrophobic and van der Waals forces.

Liu et al. [49] have also expressed the domain III of wild type HSA (wtHSAd3), which is a peptide with two known anesthetic binding sites, and a site-directed mutant of domain III (Y411Wd3) in a yeast expression system. The binding properties of halothane and propofol were examined by methods of ITC, hydrogen exchange, and fluorometry. Truncation of the wtHSA molecule to the isolated domain III did not significantly alter the secondary structure and the anesthetic binding characteristics (fewer binding sites), although the domain stability was considerably decreased in the order of wtHSA> Y411Wd3 > wtHSAd3 and the anesthetic binding affinity was reduced by less than 2-fold of wtHSA after truncation. Halothane bound two fragments while propofol could not bind to Y411Wd3. They speculated that the larger and bulky tryptophan residue sterically hinders the access of propofol to the Tyr-411 site.

2.8. Computer Simulation

More recently, binding of anesthetics to a protein has been made by computer simulation techniques [50,51]. Regarding serum albumin, in contrast with many reports on the anesthetic binding by means of various kinds of physicochemical measurements, only Seto et al. [52] have reported the difference in noble gas binding to HSA between nonimmobilizers (helium and neon) and anesthetics (argon, krypton, and xeon) by using computational docking simulation. The affinity difference between anesthetics and nonimmobilizers in an enflurane-binding site of HSA, which is known as a second binding site of propofol and has less polar nature, was studied. Their computational calculations showed that anesthetic noble gases bind to the enflurane-binding site while nonimmobilizer noble gases bind to different sites. Examining the contributions of van der Waals energy and solvent-effect energy of a noble gas at the enflurane-binding site to the total binding energy, it was found that the binding of anesthetic noble gases is dominated by van der Waals energy while nonimmobilizer noble gases is dominated by solvent-effect energy. They indicated that the binding site preferences of anesthetics and nonimmobilizer can account for their pharmacological differences and van der Waals dominance is required for anesthetic binding.

3. STRUCTUALANALYSIS OF ALBUMIN-ANESTHETIC COMPLEXES

The determination of the first high-resolution crystal structure of HSA in 1992 [10] represented a significant leap forward for drug binding studies of serum albumin. HSA is a monomeric protein of 585 amino acids with a total molecular weight of 66.4 kDa. The secondary structure of HSA is 67% α-helix and entirely lacking in β-sheet. HSA contains three homogenous α-helical domains (I-III). The domains each contain ten helices and are divided into six-helix and four-helix sub-domains (A and B); the first four helices of A and B form similar anti-parallel α-helix bundles. There is a total of 17 disulfide bridges in intra-subdomain. From the crystallographic data [10,53], it was structurally revealed that HSA is a heart-shaped protein with such features. Not a few microscopic studies of drug-binding sites on HSA have been reported since the determination of the structure.

The identification of anesthetic binding sites on HSA was done by Bhattacharya et al. [54] in 2000. They showed that propofol binds at two discrete sites on HSA. Figure 9(a) demonstrates the structure of HSA complexed with propofol, which was constructed by use of the PDB data (1E7A). One propofol molecule binds in subdomain IIIA (PR1) and the other one binds in subdomain IIIB (PR2). Similarly, they also showed that halothane binds at three sites on BSA at low concentrations of around 15% of the saturated vapor pressure (2.6 mM in the aqueous solution that is in clinically relevant concentration range). The structure of HSA complexed with halothane is depicted in Figure 9(b), which was constructed by the PDB data (1E7B). Two halothane molecules (HAL1 and HAL2) bind at the interface between subdomains IIA and IIBand a third molecule (HAL3) is present in subdomain IIIA. Furthermore, they pointed out that the binding of the anesthetics to HSA causes only very minor changes in local structure.

In the same period of time, Bhattacharya et al. [55-57] also identified binding sites of medium, long-chain, monounsaturated, and polyunsaturated fatty acids on HSA and showed that these fatty acid essentially have seven binding sites on HSA although medium fatty acids bind at additional four sites. As one example of fatty acid binding to HSA, the structure of HSA complexed with palmitic acid is drawn in Figure 10(a), which was constructed by the PDB data (1E7H). Palmitic acid clearly binds at seven discrete sites on HSA: one site in sub-domain IB (FA1), one at the interface between sub-domains IA and IIA (FA2), two in IIIA (FA3 and FA4), one in IIIB (FA5), one at the interface between IIA and IIB (FA6) and one IIA (FA7). Comparing the HSA-palmitic acid complex in Figure 10(a) with the HSA-anesthetic complexes in Figure 9, it was found that the propofol binding sites PR1 and PR2 correspond to fatty acid binding sites FA3 and FA5, and the halothane binding sites of HAL1 and HAL2 correspond to FA6 and that of HAL3 does to FA3 and FA4, respectively. In addition to a lot of binding sites in the HSA-fatty acid complex, the binding of fatty acids to HSA produces great conformational changes among three domains unlike the case of the anesthetics [54]. Fatty acid binding causes domains I and III to be displaced to the left, opening up the central crevice and increasing the width of the molecule from 80 to 90 Å. The rotation of domain I relative to domain II is stabilized by the fatty acid binding at FA2 to the interface between subdomain IA and IIA. Since the half sites formed by each subdomain have to move by about 10 Å to the adjacent binding pocket, it was suggested that the binding at FA2 acts as a pin to lock the altered conformation of HSA.

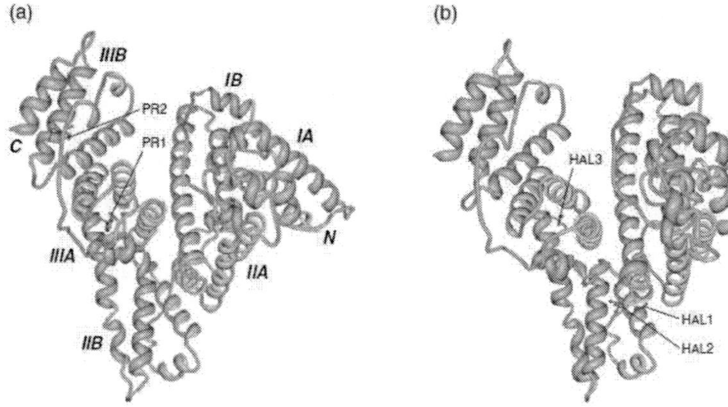

Figure 9. Structures of HSA complexed with anesthetics: (a) propofol, (b) halothane. The secondary structure of the protein, three domains I, II, III and sub-domains A and B in each domain, is shown schematically. The ligands in binding sites are represented by ball and stick models. These figures were prepared from PDB data (1E7A and 1E7B) by using MBT Protein Workshop.

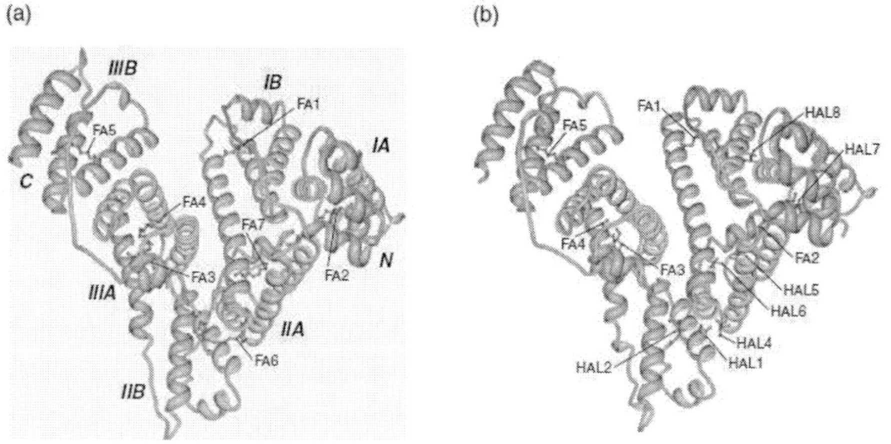

Figure 10. Structures of HSA complexed with ligands: (a) palmitic acid, (b) halothane and myristic acid. The secondary structure of the protein, three domains I, II, III and sub-domains A and B in each

domain, is shown schematically. The ligands in binding sites are represented by ball and stick models. These figures were prepared from PDB data (1E7H and 1E7C) by using MBT Protein Workshop.

At the higher halothane concentration of around 60% of the saturated vapor pressure (10.5 mM in the aqueous solution), the structure of HSA complexed with halothane was obtained in the presence of myristate. Bhattacharya et al. [54] found that there exist seven halothane-binding sites on HSA together with five myristate binding sites. Figure 10(b) shows the structure of HSA complexed with halothane and myristate (cf. PDB ID: 1E7C). Five myristate molecules bind the above-mentioned positions (FA1 to FA5). In the halothane binding, the halothane molecules HAL1 and HAL2 displaced the fatty acid FA6 while the fatty acid FA3 prevented the binding of halothane HAL3. A third halothane molecule (HAL4) binds in the trough adjacent to HAL1 and HAL2 at the interface between subdomains IIA and IIB. Two molecules (HAL5 and HAL6) bind in subdomain IIA that can also bind fatty acid FA7. Further there are two more halothane molecules. One of these (HAL7) binds at the interface between subdomains IA and IIA, of which location corresponds to the fatty acid binding site (FA8 of myristate). Finally identified the binding site (HAL8) at the interface between subdomains IA and IB was judged as a crystallographic artifact.

The structural results obtained for HSA-anesthetic and HSA-fatty acid complexes indicated that (1) propofol and halothane binding sites are amphiphilc pockets and clefts preformed on HSA, which correspond to all location of fatty-acid binding sites, (2) there are hardly changes in local structure of HSA by binding of both anesthetics at low and high concentrations. They speculated that since there is sufficient fatty acid in the blood to induce the conformational change of HSA, HAL7 might be potentially relevant pharmacologically in addition to HAL1, HAL2, and HAL3.

Ghuman et al. [58] have shown the drug-binding specificity of HSA by crystallographic analysis of many different complexes of HSA with several drugs and small-molecule toxins. They identified two primary drug-binding sites on HSA. One is a pre-formed pocket within the core of subdomain IIA, drug site 1, which corresponds to the location of FA7. Fatty acid binding markedly affects the nature of drug site 1, namely the binding alters the polarity and the volume of the site. As a results, the drug-binding specificity at drug site 1 changes. Drug site 1 mainly binds hydrophobic, bulky, hetrocyclic molecules with a centrally located negative charge (e.g. warfarin, phenylbutazone). The other exists in subdomain IIIA, drug site 2, which corresponds to the location of FA3 and FA4. Drug site 2 is smaller than site 1 and the entrance pocket is more exposed to solvent. This site binds aromatic carboxylic acids with a negative charge at one end of the molecule distal from the remaining hydrophobic structure (e.g. diazepam, ibuprofen), and it was proved to be one of main target sites of anesthetics such as propofol and halothane.

Crystallographic studies have provided a highly detailed map of binding sites of various ligand molecules including anesthetics on HSA, but they cannot provide information of the binding affinity. The problem of affinity difference in binding sites on HSA has been resolved by Simard et al [59]. They combined a ^{13}C-NMR technique with structural data complementarily and examined the binding of ^{13}C-carboxyl labeled palmitate to HSA in the absence and presence of competitor ligands to complete the correlation of NMR chemical shifts with specific structural binding sites. It was revealed that fatty-acid binding sites FA2, FA4, and FA5 are identified as high affinity sites, while sites FA1, FA3, FA6, and FA7 as low affinity sites. They explained the reason in the following way, FA2, FA4, and FA5 allow the methylene tail of the fatty acid to bind in a nearly linear conformation and the carboxyl group forms specific salt-bridge interactions with at least one basic amino acid side chain, whereas in the low affinity sites, fatty acids are obliged to bind with the methylene tail in a bent conformation that is energetically unfavorable. They also described from the affinity difference among the sites that drug site 2 (FA3 and FA4) is more susceptible to displacement by fatty acids than drug site 1 (FA7). This trend is well consistent with halothane binding to HSA at the high concentrations [54].

4. Comparative Study of Ligand Interactions

Anesthetic binding studies on BSA and HSA have exhibited that there exists a specific interaction between serum albumin and anesthetics, and X-ray crystallography identified the several binding sites of anesthetics on HSA. However, considering the following facts that most K_D (or K_I) and EC_{50} (or IC_{50}) values obtained from experiments in vitro are all in higher concentration range, anesthetics all bind the fatty-acid binding sites on serum albumin without binding the unique site to each anesthetic, no representation of pressure reversal of anesthesia for serum albumin, we wonder if anesthetic effect on serum albumin would be explainable by the specific interaction between serum albumin and anesthetics. Recently we have performed a comparative study of ligand interactions on BSA to clarify the intrinsic binding mode of anesthetics on serum albumin [60]. The comparative study was done from the three viewpoints: (1) the comparison of interaction modes of anesthetics to BSA to those of substrates or substrate analogs, what is called specific or competitive binders, (2) the comparison between thermal and volume changes by ligand binding, and (3) the comparison of the obtained macroscopic data with the structural data from X-ray crystallography, respectively.

The effect of anesthetics on serum albumin has been reported in connection with the fatty-acid binding as mentioned before. Therefore, we investigated the thermal change of BSA by binding of halothane and palmitic acid comparatively by DSC. The DSC thermograms of BSA solutions in the absence and presence of halothane and the corresponding thermograms obtained for palmitic acid are demonstrated in Figure 11, respectively. The effect of halothane appeared at concentrations of mM range, and the thermal denaturation peak of BSA shifted to the higher-temperature region and grew in a dose dependent manner.This thermal behavior of BSA for halothane was well consistent with that reported by Tanneret al. [39,40]. In the case of palmitic acid, similar peak shift to the higher-temperature region was also observed, however, the thermal behavior was significantly different from that for halothane. The temperature elevation by palmitic acid occurred at concentrations of μM range. When adding palmitic acid, bimodal thermal behavior was observed characteristically: the peak initially observed in the vicinity of 60°C decreased and another peak appeared in the higher temperature region. Further an increase in the concentration brought about a complete disappearance of the former peak and a remarkable growth of the latter peak. The denaturation temperatures and enthalpies of BSA, which were determined from the peak temperatures and areas, showed that although the binding of halothane and palmitic acid to BSA both increases the thermal stability of the BSA molecule, palmitic acid is incomparably superior in stabilization ability to halothane. Further, it was found that the peculiar thermal behavior for palmitic acid is caused at specific concentrationsat which the molar ratio of palmitic acid to BSA in the overall sample becomes ca. 4 and 7, suggesting that there exits obviously a specific interaction between the BSA and palmitic acid molecules. The stabilization of BSA by these ligands were reproduced irrespective of its forms in the pH range of 6.0 – 8.3, although the denaturation peak of BSA could not be determined because of the great peak broadening and the poor reproducibility at acidic pHs lower than 5.0 and alkaline pHs higher than 10.0.

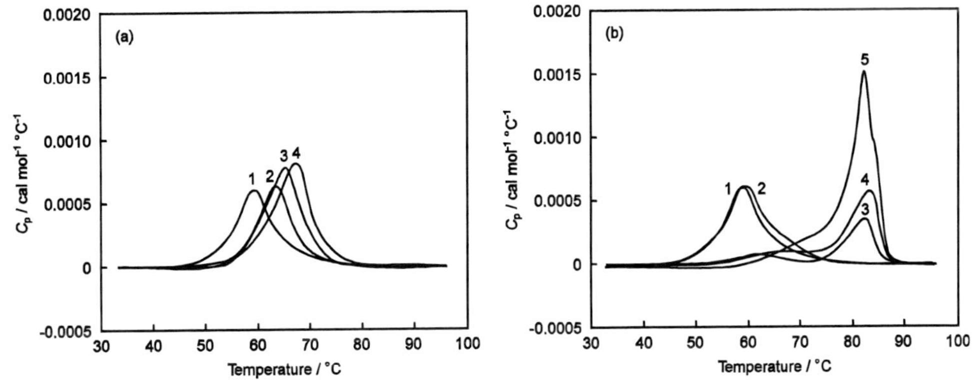

Figure 11. (a) DSC thermograms of BSA solution at pH7.0 in the absence and presence of halothane: (1) 0 mmol kg^{-1}, (2) 5, (3) 7.5, (4) 10. (b) DSC thermograms of BSA solution at pH7.0 in the absence and presence of palmitic acid: (1) 0 mmol kg^{-1}, (2) 0.01, (3) 0.05, (4) 0.1, (5) 0.2. BSA concentration is 2 mg ml^{-1}.

Ligands affect not only the thermal behavior of BSA but also the volume behavior, and pressure reversal of anesthesia is known to closely related to the volume change of biomolecules by binding of ligands. It is useful to analyze the changes in volume behavior by ligands complementarily. We next performed the comparative study of ligand effects on the volume behavior of BSA by using viscometry [60]. The pH dependence on the reduced viscosity values of BSA solutions in the absence and presence of 5 mmolalhalothane in the pH range from 2.5 to 8.3 are shown in Figure 12(a). The viscosity valuesin the absence of halothane became constant from the weak acidic pH regions to the weak alkaline pH regions, whereas at acidic pHs less than pH 4.0 they showed a stepwise viscosity increase corresponding to the E-F (pH 2.7) and F-N (pH 4.3) transitions. There was no change in the viscosity values in the vicinity of the N-B (pH 8.0) transition region. On the other hand, the viscosity values in the presence of halothane became smaller than those in the absence of halothane at all pHs measured. Similar results have been obtained by Ogli [61] for the viscosity of BSA solution saturated with gaseous halothane. The decrease in viscosity by halothane suggests that the volume of BSA in the solution shrinks by halothane, and the volume shrinkage occurs at all BSA structures irrespective of kinds of the structure. Figure 12(b) presents the pH dependence on the reduced viscosity value in the absence and presence of palmitic acid (0.15 mmolal) in the pH range from 6.0 to 8.0. The viscosity values in the presence of palmitic acid became larger than those in the absence of palmitic acid in the whole pH range measured. This viscosity increase means that the volume of BSA in the solution expands by palmitic acid in contrast with the case of halothane. By applying Einstein's equation for viscosity of hard-sphere particles in homogeneous medium, the volume change percentage of BSA by adding ligands was estimated to be -14.7% for halothane and 10.4% for palmitic acid. It turned out that halothane and palmitic acid have different effect on the volume behavior of BSA and the results of the volume behavior contrasted strikingly with those of the thermal behavior.

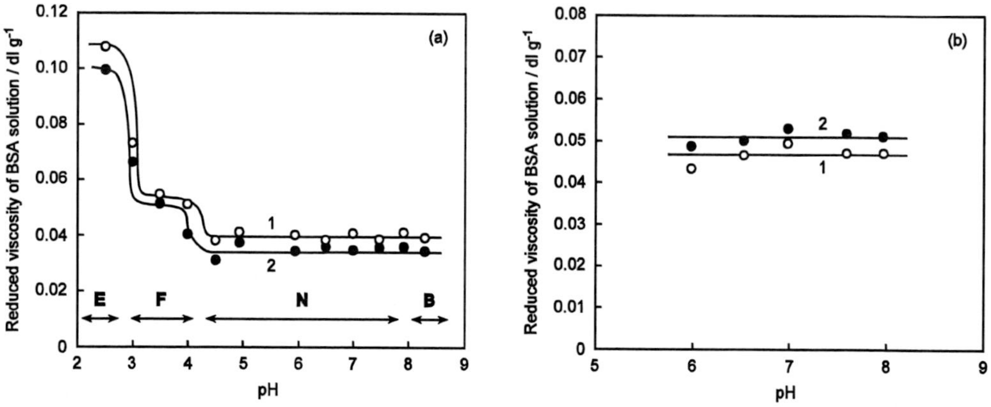

Figure 12. (a) Reduced viscosity of BSA solutions as a function of pH in the absence (1) and presence of 5-mmolal halothane (2) at 25°C.The pH region of four forms of BSA, E (expanded), F (fast), N (normal) and B (basic) is indicated in the figure. (b) Reduced viscosity of BSA solutions as a function of pH in the absence (1) and presence of 0.15-mmolal palmitic acid (2). BSA concentration is 0.5 g dl^{-1}.

BSA is about 75% identical to HSA in amino acid sequence (583 residues) and forms almost the same tertiary structure as HSA [8].As described in the previous section [54,56], the crystallographic data of the HSA-ligand complexes elucidated that halothane binds at three discrete sites on HSA at low concentrations and at seven sites at high concentrations in the presence of myristate, whereas palmitic acid binds at seven discrete sites on HSA. We inquired into the molar ratio of ligand to BSAat the effective concentration by using the overall concentrations although the binding and free concentrations between BSA and ligand at equilibrium were not determined exactly in this study. The molar ratios of effective halothane concentrations of 5 and 10 mmolal correspond to 165 and 330 moles per 1 mol of BSA while those of effective palmitic acid concentrations of 0.1 and 0.2 mmolal correspond to 3.3 and 6.6 moles, respectively. The molar ratios indicated that 50 – 100 times greater numbers of halothane molecules are required for the appearance of the ligand action on BSA whereas palmitic acid is enough for several molecules. Comparing the molar ratiosof both ligands at the effective concentrationswith the structural data, the ratio of halothane was not consistent with the binding numbers on HSA, whereas that of palmitic acid was in good agreement with the numbers. Judging from the fact that the molar ratio of halothane at the effective concentration is much larger than the concentration at the binding number, there are undoubtedly a lot of free halothane molecules in the BSA solution at the concentration. Therefore, we concluded that halothane is a very weak binder to BSA and affects BSA as a nonspecific solvent effect at the high concentrations. On the contrary, the binding mode of palmitic acid was quite different. The consistency of molar ratio and structural data suggested that the overall concentration of palmitic acid added can be substantially regarded as the binding concentration, and then there is almost no free plamitic acid in the solution at the effective concentration. Further the molar ratio at optimal stabilization observed was very close to the maximum binding number 7 from the crystallography. This fact clearly means that palmitic acid is a specific binder to BSA and stabilizes the BSA structure at the low concentrations of the binding stoichiometry.

From these comparative studies of ligand binding to BSA, we considered the difference in stabilization mechanism of the BSA structure between halothane and palmitic acid. BSA is a very hydrophilic protein and can be easily dissolved in water. Halothane and palmitic acid are both amphiphilic molecules, but palmitic acid is more hydrophobic than halothane. The difference in stabilization of BSA between ligands is closely related to that in interaction mode of a hydrophilic protein with amphiphilic ligands.We speculate that the stabilization of BSA by halothane is attributable to two factors, the predominantly hydrophilic residues on the surface and soft (less rigid) structure of BSA while the stabilization by palmitic acid is responsible for the conformational change of BSA by specific bindings of palmitic acid.

One reason for the stabilization of halothane is a great quantity of hydrophilic residues on the BSA surface. Proteins keep their structural integrity by the balance between hydrophilic and hydrophobic interactions with water. Anesthetics act at the protein/water interface and interrupt the interaction between proteins and water. For a protein with predominantly hydrophobic residues on the surface, anesthetics decrease the restrictive force of water (hydrophobic hydration) and loosen the structure. On the other hand, for a protein with predominantly hydrophilic residues at the surface, anesthetics decrease the attractive force of water (electrostriction) and tighten the structure. The above situation is similar to a poor or a good solvent in polymer chemistry. Water is repulsive to hydrophobic solutes and becomes a poor solvent, however, water is strongly attractive to hydrophilic solutes and becomes a good solvent.In a good solvent, a polymer chain is expanded, while in a poor solvent, the chain is contracted. The thermal and volume behavior of BSA in the presence of halothane suggests that the environment seems to be a poor solvent for BSA. Furthermore, since the volume of the hydrophobic interaction in water is negative [62], the effect of the hydrophobic part of anesthetic molecules on the hydrophobic residues of BSA may also contribute to the volume decrease of BSA in addition to the nonspecific solvent effect.

Another reason is the rigidity of the BSA molecule. The rigidity of a protein can be estimated from its compressibility in the aqueous solution. Gekko et al. [63,64] have examined the adiabatic compressibilities of dozens of globular proteins in water by methods of sound velocity and density measurements and classified the proteins into hard and soft categories.Theyalso revealed the correlation between the compressibility and the structural factors affecting the compressibility such as the molecular size, hydrophobicity, secondary structure, etc. of a protein.From their studies, it was found that BSA has a considerably high compressibility value, namely BSA is a very soft protein. BSA contains high-percentage of α-helix structure. The α-helix-rich proteins are known to be highly compressible [64]. Although the compressibility of α-helix itself is negligibly small [65,66], the packing of α-helix to surrounding hydrophobic region becomes insufficient due to the bulky structure, and the insufficient packing may make the compressibility of a protein increase. This indicates that it is possible for a part of α-helix in a protein to act as one of dynamic domain, and the structure of α-helixtends to soften the protein structure. Therefore, the shrinkage of BSA by halothane may result from the soft structure due to the large α-helix content.

Whereas, in the case of palmitic acid, as revealed from the structural analysis for HSA [56,57], binding of fatty acids to HSA produces the conformational change: domains I and III relative to the center domain II rotate. As mentioned in the previous section, recent studies of ^{13}C-NMR [59] and molecular dynamic simulation [67] exhibited that fatty acid binding sites FA2, FA4, and FA5 are identified as high affinity sites, while sites FA1, FA3, FA6, and FA7 as low affinity sites. Therefore, a few molecule of palmitic acid occupy the binding site of BSA, probably high affinity sites including at the interface of sub-domains IA and IIA (FA2), the conformational change of BSA from a native state to a transition state occurs, and the structure of BSA becomes thermally stable. Abrupt change in the thermal behavior in the vicinity of the molar ratio of 4 shown in Figure 11(b) may be in good agreement with the above behavior. Further increase in palmitic acid concentration brings about the greater stabilization, and when seven molecules of palmitic acid occupy all the binding sites, the maximum stabilization effect appears. Concerning the volume behavior of BSA in the presence of palmitic acid, we may say simultaneously that the conformational change due to the binding of palmitic acid produces an increase in volume of BSA [56] although the BSA structure becomes more rigid. This behavior is in accord with the fact revealed from the drug-binding study on HSA by X-ray structural analysis [58] that the binding of fatty acids increases the volume of drug site 1. We speculate that the transformation may be accompanied with a volume increase. This stabilization mechanism of palmitic acid forms a striking contrast to that of halothane.

CONCLUSION

Serum albumin is a multifunctional protein and has a number of cavities that can bind a wide array of amphiphilic hormones, metabolites, and pharmaceuticals. It has become one of the best-studied models of anesthetic binding in background of recent prosperity of a protein receptor theory of anesthesia. Various kinds of physicochemical measurements found out evidence of specific interaction between serum albumin and anesthetics. Among the measurements of X-ray structural analysis played a significant roll for the binding-site determination. However, the effective concentration of anesthetics on serum albumin showed higher values unlike other specific drugs for the albumin, indicating that anesthetics bind the sites on the albumin with much weaker interaction. Moreover, the volume behavior of serum albumin induced by anesthetic binding, which is not be paid attention at all in the above binding studies though, is not necessary in accord with a direction of pressure reversal of anesthesia. Since the volume change of a protein by anesthetics is thermodynamically related to the pressure dependence of K_D, the volume shrinkage of BSA by binding of halothane means that pressure promotes the binding of halothane to BSA, that is, pressure synergizes the anesthetic action, not antagonizes the action. This fact seems to lead to a conclusion that serum albumin is not relevant to the molecular mechanism of anesthesia. On the other hand, our comparative study indicated good correlation between the molar ratio of palmitic acid to BSA at effective concentrations in thermodynamic data and the binding numbers of palmitic acid to HSA from the structural data, confirming that a long-chain fatty acid is a specific binder to serum albumin. We think that the mechanism of serum-albumin response by various ligands including strong binders (competitors) and weak binder (anesthetics) depends on the nature of the protein and interaction modes of the ligands to the protein. The relation between binding specificity and binding affinity among ligands is ambiguous in anesthetic studies described in this chapter because there are opinions such that large-scale physicochemical changes are not necessary for anesthetic effects that take place within many types of proteins and the effect of single point mutation in a protein causes a significant modulation of the anesthetic effect. However, whenconsidering the following facts obtained for serum albumin that any anesthetics do not have a unique binding site on serum albumin and all bind the fatty-acid binding at high concentrations, the interaction modes of anesthetics are strikingly different from those of fatty acids, and anesthetic effect on serum albumin is not antagonized by pressure, we speculate that the binding bythe nonspecific weak interaction such as a solvent effect to a protein is an intrinsic interaction mode of anesthetics and the anesthetic sensibility of serum albumin is attributable to hydrophilicity of the protein surface and rigidity of the protein structure.

REFERENCES

[1] Miller, K. W. The nature of the site of general anesthesia. *Int. Rev. Neurobiol.* 1985, 27, 1-61.

[2] Trudell, J. R. Role of membrane fluidity in anesthetic action. In: Aloia, R. C., Curtain,C. C., Gordon, L. M., editors. *Drug and Anesthetic Effects on Membrane Structure and Function.* New York: Wiley-Liss; 1991; pp. 1-14.

[3] Franks, N. P.; Lieb, W. R. Where do general anesthetics act? *Nature* 1978, 274, 339-342.

[4] Franks, N. P.; Lieb, W. R. Molecular mechanisms of general anaesthesia, *Nature* 1982, 300, 487-493.

[5] Franks, N. P.; Lieb, W. R. Molecular and cellular mechanisms of general anaesthesia, *Nature* 1994, 367, 607-614.

[6] Aoki, K.; Foster, J. F. Electrophoretic behavior of bovine plasma albumin at low pH, *J. Am. Chem. Soc.* 1957, 79, 3385-3398.

[7] Foster, J. F. Some aspect of the structure and conformational properties of serum albumin. In: Rosenoer, V. M., Oratz, M., Rothschild M. A., editors, *Albumin Structure, Function and Uses.* Oxford: Pergamon Press; 1977; pp.53-84.

[8] Peters Jr., T. Serum albumin, *Advan. Protein Chem.* 1985, 37, 161-245.

[9] Carter, D. C.; Ho, J. X. Structure of serum albumin. *Adv. Protein Chem.* 1994, 45, 153-203.

[10] He, X. M.; Carter, D. C. Atomic structure and chemistry of human serum albumin. *Nature* 1992, 358, 209-215.

[11] Ho, J. X.; Holowachuk, E. W.; Norton, E. J.; Twigg, P. D.; Carter, D. C. X-ray and primary structure of horse serum albumin (Equuacaballus) at 0.27-nm resolution. *Eur. J. Biochem.* 1993, 215, 205-212.

[12] Wetlaufer, D. B.; Lovrien, R. Induction of reversible structural changes in proteins by nonpolar substances. *J. Biol. Chem.* 1964, 596-603.

[13] Balasubramanian, D.; Wetlaufer, D. B. Reversible alteration of the structure of globular proteins by anesthetic agents, *Proc. Natl. Acad. Sci. USA* 1966, 55, 762-765.

[14] Lassberg, L. H.; Hedley-Whyte, J. Halothane solubility in blood and solutions of plasma proteins: effects of temperature, protein composition and hemoglobin concentration. *Anesthesiology* 1970, 52, 351-356.

[15] Pang, Y. C.; Reid, P. E.; Brooks, D. E. Solubility and distribution of halothane in human blood. *Br. J. Anaesth.* 1980, 52, 851-861.

[16] Mashimo, T.; Suezaki, Y.; Ueda, I. Anesthetic-protein interaction: suppression of dye binding and limitation of applicability of the Scatchard plot. *Physiol. Chem. Phys.* 1982, 14, 543-551.

[17] Mashimo, T.; Kamaya, H.; Ueda, I. Anesthetic-protein interaction: surface potential of bovine serum albumin estimated by a pH-sensitive dye. *Mol. Pharmacol.* 1986, 29, 149-154.

[18] Yoshida, T.; Inagaki, H.; Kamaya, H.; Ueda, I. Two types of protein hydration measured by dielectric dispersion in the gigahertz region, and effects of anesthetics. *J. Phys. Chem. B* 2001, 105, 256-260.

[19] Ueda, I.; Mashimo, T. Anesthetic expand partial molal volume of lipid-free protein dissolved in water: electrostriction hypothesis. *Physiol. Chem. Phys.* 1982, 14, 157-164.

[20] Yamanaka, M.; Kaneshina, S.; Kamaya, H.; Ueda. I. Volumetric study on the protein-anesthetic binding. *Colloids Surf. B: Biointerf.* 2001, 22, 23-29.

[21] Eckenhoff, R. G.; Johansson, J. S. Molecular interactions between inhaled anesthetics and proteins. *Pharmacol. Rev.* 1997, 49, 343-367.

[22] Dubois, B. W.; Evers, A. S. ^{19}F-NMR spin-spin relaxation (T_2) method for characterizing volatile anesthetic binding to proteins. Analysis of isoflurane binding to serum albumin. *Biochemistry* 1992, 31, 7069-7076.

[23] Dubois, B. W.; Cherian, S. F.; Evers, A. S. Volatile anesthetics compete for common binding sites on bovine serum albumin: a ^{19}F-NMR study. *Proc. Natl. Acad. Sci. USA* 1993, 90, 6478-6482.

[24] Xu, Y.; Tang, P.; Firestone, L; Zhang, T. T. ^{19}F nuclear magnetic resonance investigation of stereoselective binding of isoflurane to bovine serum albumin. *Biophys. J.* 1996, 70, 532-538.

[25] Yoshida, T.; Tanaka, M.; Mori, Y.; Ueda, I. Negative entropy of halothane binding to protein: ^{19}F-NMR with a novel cell. *Biochim. Biophys. Acta* 1997, 1334, 117-122.

[26] Tanford C. *The hydrophobic effect: formation of micelles and biological membranes.* New York: John Wiley and Sons; 1980.

[27] Seelig, J.; Ganz, P. Nonclassical hydrophobic effect in membrane binding equilibria. *Biochemistry* 1991, 30, 9354-9359.

[28] Shikii, K.; Sakurai, S.; Utsumi, H.; Seki, H.; Tashiro, M. Application of the ^{19}F-NMR technique to observe binding of the general anesthetic halothane to human serum albumin. *Anal. Sci.* 2004, 20, 1475-1477.

[29] Eckenhoff, R. G.; Shuman, H. Halothan binding to soluble proteins determined by photoaffinity labeling. *Anesthesiology* 1993, 79, 96-106.

[30] Bosterling, B.; Trevor, A.; Trudell, J. R. Binding of halothane free radicals to fatty acids following UV radiation. *Anesthesiology* 1982, 56, 380-384.

[31] Eckenhoff, R. G.; Tanner, J. W. Differential halothane binding and effects on serum albumin and myoglobin. *Biophys. J.* 1998, 75, 477-483.

[32] Bright, D. P.; Adham, S. D.; Lemaire, L. C. J.; Benavides, R.; Gruss, M.; Taylor G. W.; Smith, E. H.; Franks, N. P. Identification of anesthetic binding sites on human serum albumin using a novel etomidatephotolabel. *J. Biol. Chem.* 2007, 282, 12038-12047.
[33] Johansson, J. S.; Eckenhoff, R. G.; Dutton, P. L. Binding of halothane to serum albumin demonstrated using tryptophan fluorescence, *Anesthesiology* 1995, 83, 316-324.
[34] Johansson, J. S. Binding of the volatile anesthetic chloroform to albumin demonstrated using tryptophan fluorescence quenching. *J. Biol. Chem.* 1997, 272, 17961-17965.
[35] Takehara, K.; Morinaga, Y.; Nakashima, S.; Matsuoka, S.; Kamaya, H.; Ueda, I. Classification of the binding modes in bovine serum albumin using terminally substituted alkane analogues. *Anal. Sci.* 2006, 22, 1571-1575.
[36] Takehara, K.; Yuki, K.; Shirasawa, M.; Yamasaki, S.; Yamada, S. Binding properties of hydrophobic molecules to human serum albumin studies by fluorescence titration. 2009, 25, 115-120.
[37] Eckenhoff, R. G. Do specific or nonspecific interactions with proteins underlie inhalational anesthetic action? *Mol. Pharmacol.* 1998, 54, 610-615.
[38] Chiou, J.-S.; Ueda, I. Ethanol unfolds firefly luciferase while competitive inhibitors antagonize unfolding: DSC and FT-IR analysis. *J. Pharm. Biomed. Anal.* 1994, 12, 969-975.
[39] Tanner, J. W.; Liebman, P. A.; Eckenhoff, R. G. Volatile anesthetics alter protein stability. *Toxicol. Lett.* 1998, 100-101, 387-391.
[40] Tanner, J. W.; Eckenhoff, R. G.; Liebman, P. A. Halothane, an inhalational anesthetic agent, increases folding stability of serum albumin. *Biochim. Biophys. Acta*1999, 1430, 46-56.
[41] Ueda, I.; Yamanaka, M. Titration calorimetry of anesthetic-protein interaction: negative enthalpy of binding and anesthetic potency. *Biophys. J.* 1997, 72, 1812-1817.
[42] Sawas, A. H.; Pentyala, S. N.; Rebecchi, M. J. Binding of volatile anesthetics to serum albumin: measurements of enthalpy and solvent contributions. *Biochemistry* 2004, 43, 12675-12685.
[43] Liu, R.; Meng, Q.; Xi, J.; Yang, J.; Ha, C.-E.; Bhagavan, N. V.; Eckenhoff, R. G. Comparative binding character of two general anaesthetics for sites on human serum albumin. *Biochem. J.* 2004, 380, 147-152.
[44] Liu, R.; Eckenhoff, R. G. Weak polar interactions confer albumin binding site selectivity for haloether anesthetics. *Anesthesiology* 2005, 102, 799-805.
[45] Chan, K.; Meng, Q. C.; Johansson, J. S.; Echenhoff, R. G. Low-affinity analytical chromatography for measuring inhaled anesthetic binding to isolated proteins, *Anal. Biochem.* 2002, 301, 308-313.
[46] Eckenhoff, R. G. Amino acid resolution of halothane binding sites in serum albumin, *J. Biol. Chem.* 1996, 271, 15521-15526.
[47] Eckenhoff, R. G.; Peterson, C. E.; Ha, C.-E.; Bhagavan, N. V. Inhaled anesthetic binding sites in human serum albumin. *J. Biol. Chem.* 2000, 275, 30439-30444.
[48] Liu, R.; Pidikiti, R.; Ha, C.-E.; Peterson, C. E.; Bhagavan, N. V.; Eckenhoff, R. G. The role of electrostatic interactions in human serum albumin binding and stabilization by halothane. *J. Biol. Chem.* 2002, 277, 36373-36379.
[49] Liu, R.; Yang, J.; Ha, C.-E.; Bhagavan, N. V.; Eckenhoff, R. G. Truncated human serum albumin retains general anesthetic binding activity. *Biochem. J.* 2005, 388, 39-45.

[50] Streiff, J. H.; Jones, K. A. Volatile anesthetic binding is influenced by solvent and aliphatic residues. *J. Chem. Inf. Model.* 2008, 48, 2066-2073.
[51] Vemparala, S.; Domene, C.; Klein, M. L. Computational studies on the interactions of inhalation anesthetics with proteins. *Acc. Chem. Res.* 2010, 43, 103-110.
[52] Seto, T.; Isogai, H.; Ozaki, M.; Nosaka, S. Noble gas binding to human serum albumin using docking simulation: nonimmobilizer and anesthetics bind to different sites. *Anesth. Analg.* 2008, 107, 1223-1228.
[53] Sugio, S.: Kashima, A.: Mochizuki, S.; Noda, M.; Kobayashi, K. Crystal sturucture of human serum albumin at 2.5 Å resolution. *Protein Eng.* 1999, 12, 439-446.
[54] Bhattacharya, A. A.; Curry, S.; Franks, N. P. Binding of the general anesthetic propofol and halothane to human serum albumin. *J. Biol. Chem.* 2000, 275, 38731-38738.
[55] Curry, S.; Brick, P.; Franks, N. P. Fatty acid binding to human serum albumin: new insight from crystallographic studies, *Biochim. Biophys. Acta* 1999, 1441, 131-140.
[56] Bhattacharya, A. A.; Grüne, T.; Curry, S. Crystallographic analysis reveals common modes of binding of medium and long-chain fatty acids to human serum albumin. *J. Mol. Biol.* 2000, 303, 721-732.
[57] Petitpas, I.; Grüne, T.; Bhattacharya, A. A.; Curry, S. Crystal structures of human serum albumin complexed with monounsaturated and polyunsaturated fatty acids. *J. Mol. Biol.* 2001, 314, 955-960.
[58] Ghuman, J.; Zunszain, P. A,;Petitpas, I.; Bhattacharya, A. A.; Otagiri, M; Curry, S. Structural basis of the drug-binding specificity of humen serum albumin. *J. Mol. Biol.* 2005, 353, 38-52.
[59] Simard, J. R.; Zunszain, P. A,; Hamilton, J. A.; Curry, S. Location of high and low affinity fatty acid binding sites on human serum albumin revealed by NMR drug-competition analysis. *J. Mol. Biol.* 2006, 361, 336-351.
[60] Nishimoto, M.; Komatsu, U.; Tamai, N.; Yamanaka, M.; Kaneshina, S.; Ogli, K.; Matsuki, H. A comparative study on specific and nonspecific interactions in bovine serum albumin: thermal and volume effects of halothane and palmitic acid. *Colloid Polym. Sci.* 2009, 287, 979-989.
[61] Ogli, K. Halothane decreases the viscosity of bovine serum albumin (BSA) solution, In: Urban, B. W., Barann M., editors, *Molecular and Basic Mechanisms of Anesthesia*, Berlin: Pabst Scientific Publishers; 2002; pp. 36-39.
[62] Ben-Naim, A. *Hydrophobic Interactions*. New York: Plenum Press; 1980; Chapter 5.
[63] Gekko, K.; Noguchi, H. Compressibility of globular proteins in water at 25°C. *J. Phys. Chem.* 1979, 83, 2706-2714.
[64] Gekko, K.; Hasegawa, Y. Compressibility-structure relationship of globular proteins, *Biochemistry* 1986, 25, 6563-6571.
[65] Takekiyo, T.; Imai, T.; Kato, M.; Taniguchi, Y. Understanding high pressure stability of helical conformation of oligopeptides and helix bundle proten, high pressure FT-IR and RISM theoretical studies, *Biochim. Biophys. Acta*2006, 1764, 355-363.
[66] Takekiyo, T.; Takeda, N.; Isogai, Y.; Kato, M.; Taniguchi, Y. Pressure stability of the α-helix structure in a de novo designed protein $(\alpha\text{-I-}\alpha)_2$ studied by FTIR spectroscopy, *Biopolymers* 2007, 85, 185-188.
[67] Fujiwara, S.; Amisaki, T. Identification of High Affinity fatty acid binding sites on human serum albumin by MM-PBSA method, *Biophys. J.* 2008, 94, 92-103.

In: Serum Albumin: Structure, Functions and Health Impact ISBN: 978-1-62100-231-4
Editors: R. J. Alekseev and A. L. Rebane

Chapter 3

MICROPARTICULATE DRUG DELIVERY SYSTEMS BASED ON SERUM ALBUMIN

Florence Edwards-Lévy*
Institute of Molecular Chemistry of Reims, Faculty of Pharmacy of Reims,
University of Reims Champagne-Ardenne, France

ABSTRACT

Drug delivery systems are developed to improve the efficacy, bioavailability and pharmacokinetic properties of therapeutically active molecules. These systems have to meet precise requirements, like biocompatibility and biodegradability. Furthermore, the active molecule has to be bound and protected by the system until it reaches a physiological target, and then the system is able to release the molecule in a controlled manner. The release kinetics of the bioactive molecule by an ideal delivery system is designed for an optimized therapeutic effect in vivo, and this kinetics is synchronized with the degradation kinetics of the system itself.

Microparticulate drug delivery systems, i.e. microcapsules and microspheres, present an interesting surface-to-volume ratio, favoring exchange phenomena between their load and the physiological environment after administration. The interactions and release kinetics of various molecules with microparticles can be precisely controlled by the size of the particles, and by the parameters of the process used to produce them. Many methods are now developed to produce microparticles, based on physical, physico-chemical or chemical processes. Easily available and often biocompatible, biopolymers play an increasing role among the materials available to constitute the frame of microparticles.

In this context, serum albumin is an emerging biopolymer presenting very attractive properties for its use as a constitutive material for microparticulate drug delivery systems. This endogeneous macromolecule, already used in human health for the treatment of various diseases by different routes, is perfectly biocompatible and biodegradable. Albumin is known for its binding properties towards various xenobiotics, and for its solubilizing properties towards hydrophobic compounds. Moreover, albumin presents physicochemical properties like high solubility in water, low viscosity in solution,

*E-mail: Florence.edwards@univ-reims.fr

interfacial properties, denaturation upon heating, which can be very useful in encapsulation processes. Furthermore, this protein bears many functional groups available for chemical modifications needed for encapsulation by chemical methods.

This paper reviews the methods used to produce microparticles from serum albumin for drug delivery purposes. The methods based on physical, physico-chemical and chemical processes will be described, as well as studies dealing with the properties of the resulting microparticles.

INTRODUCTION

Serum albumin, the most abundant plasma protein, is a readily available, non-toxic, non-antigenic if of human origin, biocompatible and biodegradable polymer. This endogeneous protein is known for its binding properties towards various xenobiotics, and for its solubilizing properties towards hydrophobic compounds. Albumin presents physicochemical properties like high solubility in water, low viscosity in solution, interfacial properties, denaturation upon heating, which can be very useful in encapsulation processes. Furthermore, this protein bears many functional groups available for chemical modifications needed for encapsulation by chemical methods. For all of these reasons, serum albumin is widely used to prepare microparticles [1; 2].

The main purposes of drug delivery systems are the protection of fragile molecules against degradation, the local release of drugs to avoid systemic side effects, the sustained drug release avoiding multiple administrations and increasing patient compliance, drug release controlled by a local environment (pH, temperature, or magnetic field for example), the increase of drug solubility, and the global improvement of drug bioavailability.

Microparticulate drug delivery systems [3-5] can be divided in two categories depending on their internal structure (figure 1). Microspheres are spherical matrices with a homogeneous or heterogeneous solid content, whereas microcapsules are vesicular structures with a content of various nature surrounded by a membrane. The membrane of a microcapsule releases the content by diffusion, or upon destruction, or is intended to keep the content enclosed.

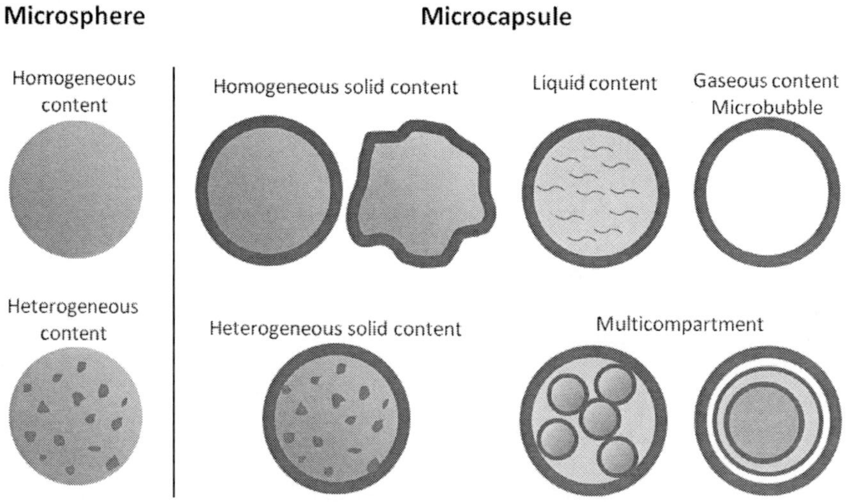

Figure 1. Schematic morphologies of microspheres and microcapsules.

Among the different drug delivery systems, microcapsules and microspheres offer several advantages. Microparticles present an interesting surface-to-volume ratio, favoring exchanges between the delivery system and the local environment. This discrete system is spreadable over a defined surface for local delivery, avoiding the release of the drug in an unwanted site [6]. Microparticles can be injected in the bloodstream, their size being the decisive factor for their biodistribution after injection. Small microspheres (less than 3 μm) are taken up by the reticuloendothelial system and accumulate in the liver and the spleen. These small microspheres accumulate in solid tumors too, due to the enhanced penetration and retention (EPR) effect [7]. They can be phagocytized by cells, and potentiate the therapeutic effect of drugs by increasing their cellular uptake. Larger microparticles (> 15 μm) are blocked in the capillary bed of the lungs [8], and this efficient lung targeting can be used to deliver drugs, or for imaging. Microparticles of a higher diameter can be injected in an artery near a tumor, for embolization [9], or its variants, i.e. chemoembolization [10](emboles loaded with antitumoral drug) and radioembolization [11](emboles loaded with radionuclides). Microbubbles, i.e. microscopic air bubbles trapped within a membrane, can be used for contrast in medical ultrasonography [12], for vascular gene delivery [13], or for a non invasive imaging of acute inflammation after microbubble phagocytosis by inflammatory cells [14]. Albumin possesses the property of accumulating in malignant and inflamed tissues when in solution in the bloodstream [2]. In the form of a solid particle, the system can acquire targeting properties, by loading with magnetite and guiding through an extracorporeal magnet [15], or by grafting specific ligands on the particle surface [12]. Other routes are being studied for the administration of albumin microparticles. Intramuscular injections of drug-loaded microparticles of various size ranges are studied for local slow release of drugs [16]. Intracavitary [17] or intratumoral [18] injections of antitumoral drugs entrapped into albumin microparticles improve the treatment. Intraarticular injection of microspheres loaded with anti-inflammatory drugs is effective in improving the retention of the drug in the joint cavity for a longer effect [19]. The drug-loaded particles may also be implanted at the site where the drug will be released [20-24]. Mucoadhesive properties can be given to the particle surface, leading to interesting long-lasting local delivery systems for the nasal route [25] or for ocular preparations [26]. Local delivery of antibiotics by topical administration of microparticles can solve the dilemma of maintaining a high local antibiotic concentration while avoiding systemic side effects [27]. Particles with specific aerodynamic properties and low density can be developed for local lung treatments [28]. Studies can be found in the literature concerning the use of albumin microparticles by the oral route [29; 30]. According to the goal, different kinds of formulations can be produced using microparticles. For example they can be administered as free powders in dry powder inhalers for lung treatment, as suspensions for the parenteral or transdermal route, or incorporated in capsules or tablets for the oral route [31]. For drug loading, two ways are possible: during the preparation of the microparticles (for most studies available in the literature), or after the formation of the particles, by impregnation into the polymer matrix [24], or by adsorption or fixation onto the surface [17]. Serum albumin by itself does not provide any sustained release properties, and has to be cross-linked or stabilized using various methods in order to achieve sustained or controlled release properties [26]. This non-exhaustive review will present a panel of different technologies developed for the preparation of microparticles from albumin, based on physical, physico-chemical or chemical processes. The studies dealing with serum albumin will be mainly exposed. Due to structural similarities, in some studies egg white albumin is being used instead of serum albumin and examples of these studies will be presented too.

Serum Albumin for the Preparation of Microparticulate Drug Delivery Systems

-Physical Methods

Emulsification-thermal denaturation of albumin solutions is one of the most used methods to prepare albumin-based microparticles [27]. The preparation procedure first involves an emulsification step of the aqueous solution of albumin containing the drug, in an oily phase (figure 2). After homogenization of the emulsion, a volume of heated oil is added and mixed to the emulsion. The heating treatment creates intermolecular disulfide bridges between serine residues of adjacent protein chains [32], leading to insolubilization of the protein in the form of microspheres. The reversible unfolding of the protein begins at 50°C, and above 65°C this unfolding gives an easy access to the formation of disulfide bridges [27]. The effect is more pronounced when the temperature is above 100°C, and increases as the heating is prolonged. Some variations can be found in the literature regarding the method used to divide the aqueous phase in small droplets prior to the heating step. For example emulsification using a glass membrane with controlled pore size was found to produce particles with a narrower size distribution than with a classical stirrer [33]. The heating method can also be varied, and the use of microwaves produced smaller microspheres in a shorter time [34]. Kramer first suggested this method for delivery of anticancer drugs and demonstrated that drug-containing microspheres presenting a diameter of 0.5-1.2 μm were phagocytized by different cell lines [35; 36]. Various anticancer drugs were then encapsulated by this method [37-40]. Other drugs resisting to elevated temperatures could also be encapsulated using this method, and good results were obtained with drugs such as antibiotics [27; 41], steroids [42; 43], or propranolol [44].

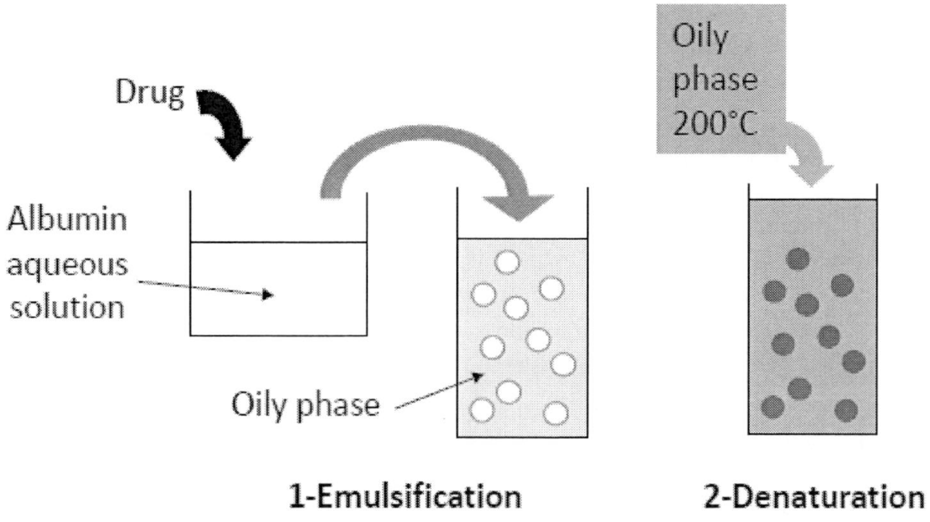

Figure 2. Preparation of albumin microspheres by the emulsification-thermal denaturation method.

The thermal denaturation method is currently applied to the delivery of radionuclides for diagnostic or therapeutic purposes. Microspheres made of heat-denaturated albumin are available as kits for the extemporaneous preparation of ^{99m}Tc-labelled particles used for lung imaging (figure 3)[45-47]. As an alternative to blood derived albumin, recombinant human serum albumin (rHSA) produced by yeast cells has been developed to overcome the risk of viral/prion contamination [48], and rHSA microspheres have been used in scintigraphic studies [49]. Heat-denaturated albumin microspheres present the advantages of possessing a monodisperse size distribution and a regular shape, as compared with macroaggregated serum albumin prepared by precipitating serum albumin with Sn(II) chloride [45; 47; 49-51]. Furthermore, their biocompatibility and biodegradability make these particles more attractive than glass microspheres or resin microspheres classically used as radionuclide carriers for radioembolization of tumors [47; 52-56]. Other inorganic compounds have been loaded in heat-denatured albumin microspheres, like gadolinium [57] for imaging, or magnetite for drug targeting [15; 32; 34; 39; 58] after the precursory studies of Widder and co-workers concerning the encapsulation of anticancer drugs in magnetically guidable albumin microspheres [59-61]. *Spray-drying* is another very popular method to produce albumin microspheres. A device is used to atomize and dry in one step a solution or suspension containing the protein and the compound to encapsulate. Atomization generates fine droplets with a large air-liquid interfacial area. Then the droplets dry very rapidly in a current of heated air. This technique produces insoluble microspheres, provided that the drying temperature allows the thermal denaturation of the protein. Otherwise, the technique has to be coupled with a chemical cross-linking step, as it will be described later, to produce non-soluble objects. The advantages of spray-drying are that the product is free of solvent residues, and the process is possible in a continuous operation. The main components of a standard spray-drying apparatus include a nozzle, a spray chamber, the air heater, a cyclone to separate the dried particles from the air, and a vessel to collect them (figure 4) [62]. Various systems are available regarding the atomization system (rotary nozzle, pressure atomization, two-fluid nozzle ...) and the direction of the spray feed materials and the drying air (co-current or counter-current). After the choice of the type of spray-dryer, parameters have to be set for the formulation of the sprayed liquid (solvent, concentration of the polymeric solution to be sprayed, presence of additives, drug/polymer ratio), and on the apparatus (drying temperature, spraying rate ...). These parameters influence the properties of the resulting particles, like aerodynamic properties (important for aerosol delivery to the lungs for example) or controlled release properties [28). Controlling the evaporation rate of water from the sprayed droplets makes possible to influence the global shape and the nanoscaled substructure of the microparticles [63; 64]. Furthermore, both water-soluble and water-insoluble drugs can be loaded in albumin microspheres by using this technique, and the whole procedure can be carried out aseptically for the preparation of particles intended to be administered parenterally [62). Various drugs have been encapsulated with albumin using this method. The encapsulation of ciprofloxacin for pulmonary delivery provided a sustained release after thermal treatment [65]. In another study, particles loaded with nicardipine presented interesting mucoadhesive properties for their use for the nasal route [66]. For parenteral administration of molecules with important side effects (Amphotericin B [67], doxorubicin [17]), their encapsulation led to an increase of the therapeutic index. Furthermore, studies on microparticles obtained by spray-drying demonstrated that the encapsulation favored the cellular uptake of some drugs (miltefosin [68], paromomycin [69]), and thus their efficacy. The technique has also been applied to the encapsulation of quantum dots (figure 5), the microspheres emitting bright fluorescence after incorporation of the quantum dots, and the polymer matrix shielding the toxicity of the fluorescent nanoparticles [70].

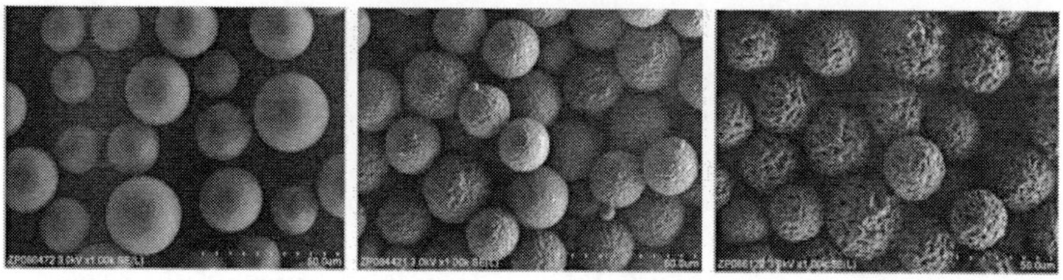

Figure 3. SEM photographs of three different batches of heat-denaturated serum albumin microspheres for radioembolization. Reprinted from Schiller E et al., Nuclear Medicine and Biology 2008; 35(2):227-232, with permission from Elsevier.

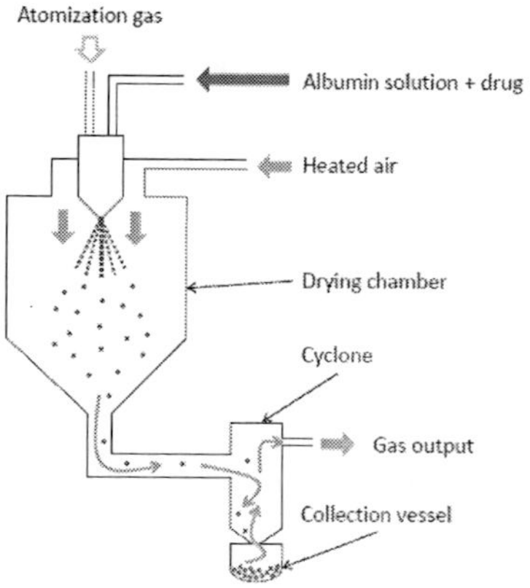

Figure 4. Preparation of albumin microspheres by the spray-drying method (co-current).

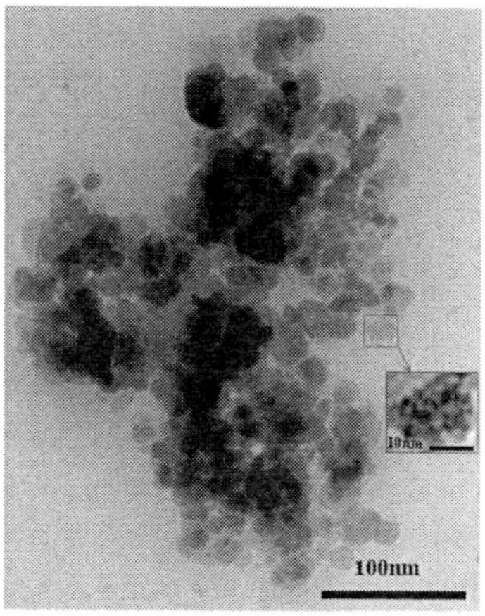

Figure 5. TEM image of spray-dried serum albumin microspheres containing quantum dot. Reprinted with permission from M. Chu et al., Nanotechnology 2006; 17(6):1791-1796, IOP Publishing Ltd. http://dx.doi.org/10.1088/0957-4484/17/6/041.

Aqueous solutions containing albumin can be divided in very fine and monodisperse droplets using a *supercritical-assisted atomization (SAA) process* [31; 27; 71]. This technique has been successfully tested for the micronization of some pharmaceutical compounds, and was recently proposed by Reverchon and coworkers for the preparation of microparticulate drug delivery systems [31]. This green process presents the advantages of avoiding the use of high temperatures or solvents difficult to remove, and produces small (0.1 to 5 μm) microspheres with a controlled size distribution. The method is based on the solubilization of controlled quantities of supercritical carbon dioxide (SC-CO_2) in the liquid containing the matrix-forming polymer and the drug (figure 6). The mixture is delivered in a saturator, which is a high pressure vessel equipped with internal perforated walls to ensure a large contact surface between the liquid solution and SC-CO_2. The solution obtained is then sprayed through a thin injection nozzle into the precipitator, together with a controlled flow of heated nitrogen which facilitates liquid droplet evaporation [27].

The SC-CO_2 acts in the process as a co-solute, miscible to the solution to be treated, and as a pneumatic agent to atomize the solution in very fine droplets. A two-step atomization is obtained, the primary droplets produced at the outlet of the injection nozzle (pneumatic atomization) are further divided in secondary droplets by CO_2 expansion from the inside of the primary ones (decompressive atomization). Gentamicin sulfate has been successfully encapsulated in albumin heat-denaturated microspheres prepared by SAA, with high encapsulation efficiency and diffusion-controlled release of the antibiotic from the microspheres [27]. The process has been recently improved by replacing the saturator by a hydrodynamic cavitation mixer, to intensify the mixing between the liquid and SC-CO_2 [71].

A cryogenic process has been applied to the preparation of albumin microspheres, by *spray freezing into liquid nitrogen* [72]. In this method, the solution is sprayed directly through a fine nozzle into liquid nitrogen. The high pressure drop through the nozzle combined with the friction generated by passing the droplets through a liquid rather than a vapor phase result in an intense atomization of the droplets. The very fast freezing avoids protein unfolding at the interface and further particle aggregation. After lyophilization, very small, porous, low density particles can be formed, which appear to be suitable for pulmonary delivery.

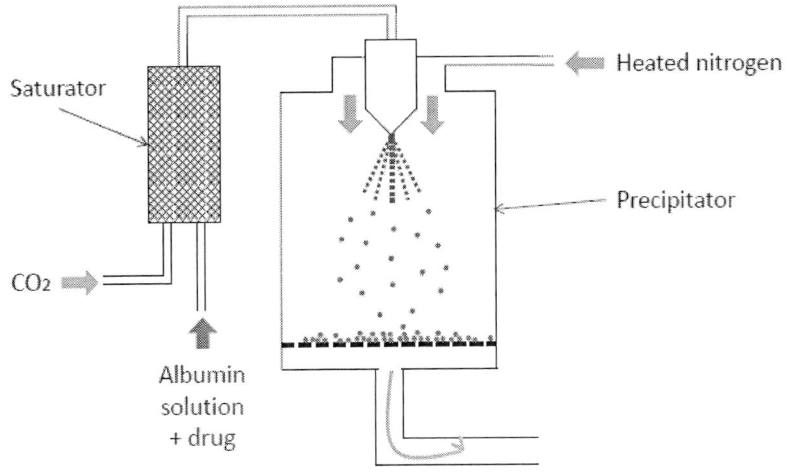

Figure 6. Preparation of albumin microspheres by the supercritical-assisted atomization process.

The *sonochemical method*, first developed by Süslick in the 90s, requires a high-intensity ultrasonic probe to produce microparticles from proteins [73-76]. Liquid-filled microcapsules with a narrow size distribution can be obtained by applying high-intensity ultrasound to a mixture of aqueous phase containing albumin, and organic solvent to encapsulate. The effect of ultrasounds both produces emulsification of the two phases, and cross-linking of protein molecules. The physical phenomenon responsible for the sonochemical process is acoustic cavitation. Ultrasounds create local pressure drops in the liquid, forming microscopic gas bubbles. These bubbles grow until they reach a maximum size. The implosive collapse of the bubbles occurs very rapidly and creates free radicals in the aqueous phase. Superoxide free radicals have been shown to be responsible for the chemical cross-linking of albumin through disulfide bonds between cysteine residues [74-76]. Avivi and Gedanken have however demonstrated that cysteine residues are not always required to form microparticles with this method [73; 77]. They managed to produce microparticles with the sonochemical process using a protein without cysteine, like streptavidin, by lowering the pH of the medium to 6. In this case, hydrophobic or thermal denaturation of the protein during the ultrasonic emulsification accounts for microsphere formation, and the lightly acidic pH helps to neutralize the carboxylate groups of the protein, thus creating a more hydrophobic environment. The sonochemical method can also be used to produce gas-filled microcapsules or microbubbles, the difference in the formation of liquid- and gas-filled microcapsules being the position of the ultrasonic probe [73; 76]. For the preparation of liquid-filled microcapsules, the organic liquid is layered over the protein solution and the probe is placed at the solvent-water interface. For air-filled microbubbles, the probe is placed at the air-water interface. The method has been explored regarding the influence of the preparation parameters on production yield and size distribution [76; 78] and on the release profile of hydrophobic compounds from the microcapsules [79]. The procedure could also be applied to the preparation of mixed proteinaceous microparticles [80]. Various active ingredients have been encapsulated by this method, including anticancer drugs (figure 7) [81; 82], antibiotics [83], or magnetite [84; 85]. The attachment of a specific peptide by electrostatic adhesion on the surface of the sonochemically-prepared particles led to systems able of tumor targeting [12].

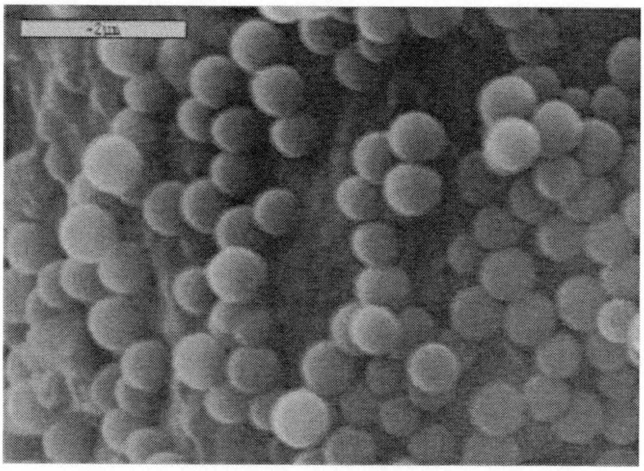

Figure 7. SEM photograph of gemcitabine-loaded serum albumin microspheres prepared sonochemically (81). Reprinted from Grinberg O et al., Acta Biomaterialia 2009; 5(8):3031-3037, with permission from Elsevier.

-Physico-Chemical Methods

Among the methods based on phase separation, *coacervation* corresponds to a desolvation phenomenon, leading to a separation into two liquid phases in the colloidal system, the more concentrated phase being the coacervate, and the diluted one is the equilibrium solution. This method has been extensively studied by Langer and co-workers to produce human serum albumin nanoparticles of controllable size by adding ethanol to an aqueous solution of the protein [86-88]. The method can also be applied to produce protein membranes around cores of micrometric sizes and of various natures, as desolvated proteins tend to deposit onto surfaces (figure 8).

Möhwald and co-workers have developed a technique to produce hollow albumin microcapsules in three steps (figure 9) successively involving desolvation of the protein onto a sacrificial core by slow addition of ethanol, chemical cross-linking of the membrane (see below), and dissolution of the core [89]. The amount of desolvated albumin can be controlled by varying the amount of ethanol used for desolvation, which in turn influences the wall thickness of the resulting microcapsules.

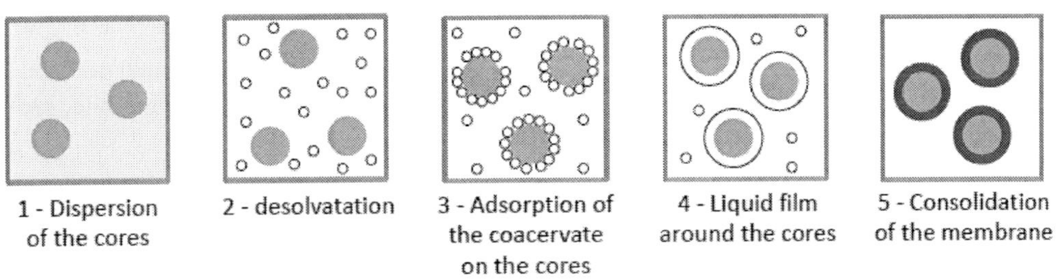

Figure 8. Preparation of microcapsules by the coacervation method.

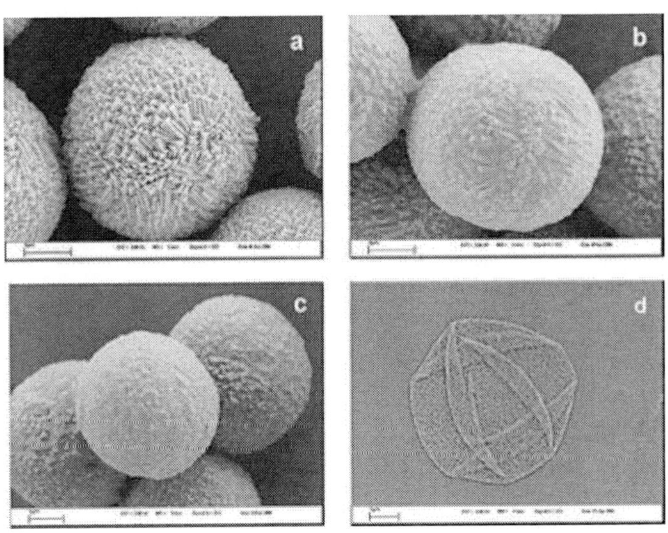

Figure 9. SEM images of (a) bare $MnCO_3$ microparticles, (b) bovine serum albumin-adsorbed $MnCO_3$ microparticles, (c) BSA-adsorbed $MnCO_3$ microparticles further cross-linked, and (d) a hollow BSA microcapsule. Scale bar: 1 μm (89). Reproduced from Zhu Y et al., Journal of Materials Chemistry 2008; 18(10):1153-1158, with permission of The Royal Society of Chemistry. http://dx.doi.org/10.1039/b714647g.

Complex coacervation is coacervation caused by the interaction of two oppositely charged colloids. Microcapsules with walls made of a protein-polysaccharide ionic association can be produced by complex coacervation [90]. A neutral complex of the two polymers forms when the pH is such that the number of positive charges on the protein matches the number of negative charges on the anionic polysaccharide. The neutral coacervate deposits on solid cores or immiscible droplets mixed to the medium. This method was first described with the system gelatin-acacia gum and applied in the famous patent on carbon-less copying paper [91]. A few studies deal with the use of albumin, associated with alginic acid [92] or with acacia gum [93] for encapsulation purposes. The coacervate resulting from the association of albumin with alginic acid was too viscous to adapt the system for microencapsulation, whereas conditions have been found for which the association of albumin with acacia gum spontaneously produced stable microgel coacervate particles of a few micrometers in diameter. Conditions influencing complex coacervation have also been studied between albumin and sulfated polysaccharides such as dextran sulfate [94] or carrageenans [95], but no applications in microencapsulation have been developed yet.

Emulsification-solvent evaporation is a method involving the preparation of a solution of the microsphere-forming polymer(s) and the drug in a volatile solvent, and further emulsification of the solution in a non-miscible phase. Evaporation of the internal phase is started upon moderate heating under low pressure. Deprived of its solvent, the protein precipitates and the microsphere is formed, entrapping the drug [96].

Another technique using solvent evaporation and involving interfacial properties of proteins was proposed by Lu et al. and produces microcapsules of a few micrometers in size and surrounded by a membrane made of a pure protein [97]. The technique consists in adding droplets of an organic solvent into a diluted buffered albumin solution. After a few minutes, the protein adsorbed onto the interface and the solvent was removed by evaporation. The stability of the resulting particles was attributed to albumin unfolding at the interface, exposing nonpolar amino side chains and making the unfolded protein less hydrosoluble than the native one.

The deposit of alternative layers of oppositely charged polyelectrolytes onto a template is called *"layer-by-layer" technique* [98], and by using spherical templates of micrometric sizes the system produces microcapsules [99-106]. This mild nanoassembly method does not involve any covalent binding and is based on the cooperative electrostatic attraction of the sequentially adsorbed polyanions and polycations (figure 10).

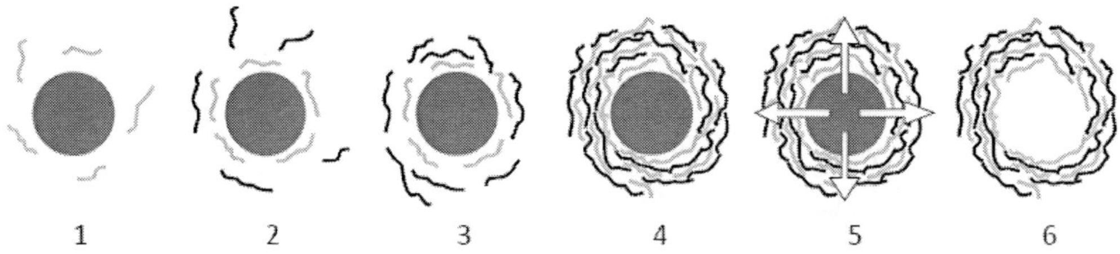

Figure 10. Preparation of microcapsules by the layer-by-layer method. (1) Adsorption of a first layer of polyelectrolyte, charge opposed to the charge of the core, (2) and (3) adsorption of the second layer, polyelectrolyte charged like the core, (4) multilayered membrane around the core, (5) redissolution of the sacrificial core, (6) hollow microcapsule.

The thickness and permeability of the nanoporous membranes of polyelectrolyte microcapsules can be adjusted by controlling the number of layers as well as the environmental conditions. The whole process can be easily monitored by measuring the zeta potential of the particles at each stage of the assembly and adjusting the pH for the appearance of adequate charges on the particles and on the polymer.

In the studies of An and co-workers, the membrane is formed by the association of albumin and phospholipid layers [101-103; 105], but other polymers can be associated to albumin. The internal solid microparticles can be redissolved after the edification of the multilayered membrane (sacrificial template). In other cases, the solid particle onto which the multilayered membrane was constructed represents the compound to be encapsulated, like albumin microbubbles decorated by electrostatically linked RGD-peptide for targeting [12], drug crystals for controlled release [101], or bacterial spores for protection and controlled germination [104].

-Chemical Methods

Several simple dialdehydes have been shown to form protein cross-links [107]. The most extensively used reagent is glutaraldehyde. The reaction should involve amino groups on the protein through Schiff bases; however the product formed is irreversible. Glutaraldehyde has been found to form polymers in solution, at neutral or slightly alkaline pH, and presumably it is the unsaturated polymer that cross-links the amino groups of the protein, creating a network of cross-linked protein (figure 11).

Formaldehyde can also be used as a cross-linker. Formaldehyde is not strictly a dialdehyde but is capable of reacting bifunctionally, and can form bridges between two protein molecules by a two-step reaction (figure 12)[107]. Some examples of formaldehyde cross-linked albumin microspheres can be found in the literature [108; 109].

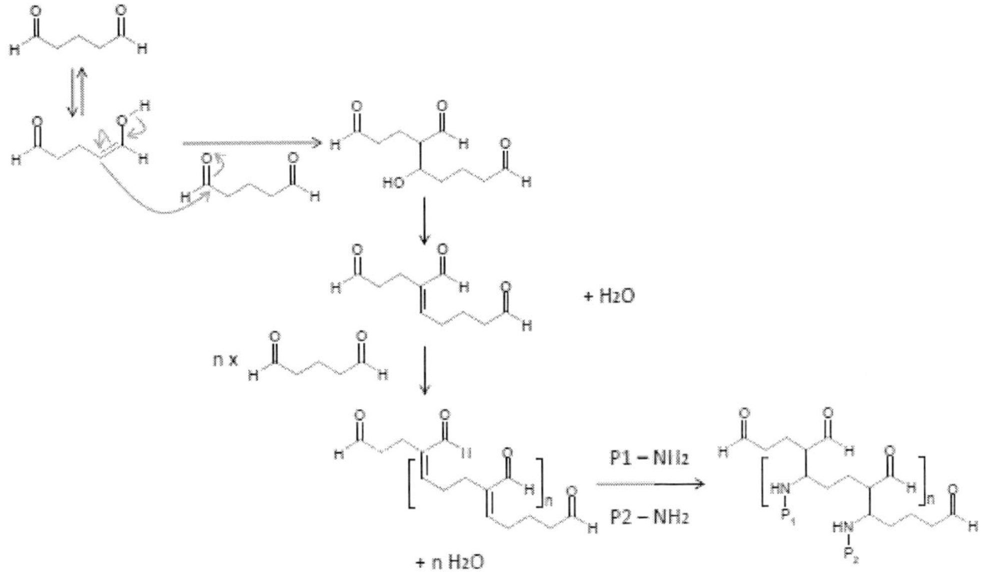

Figure 11. Polymerization of glutaraldehyde and its cross-linking reaction with proteins.

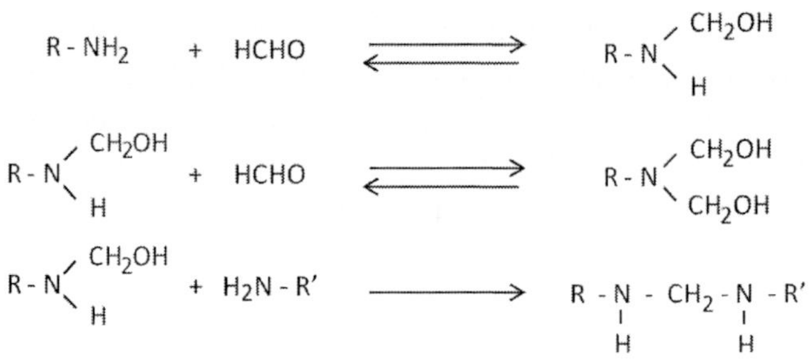

Figure 12. reaction of formaldehyde with amino groups of proteins.

The *emulsion-cross-linking method* described by Lee and co-workers is often cited as a reference for the preparation of covalently cross-linked albumin microspheres using glutaraldehyde [110]. The technique consists in dissolving the drug into an aqueous solution of albumin. The solution is emulsified in a hydrophobic phase generally consisting of cottonseed oil or its mixture with petroleum ether, and containing a surfactant for emulsion stabilization. Cross-linking is started upon addition of an aqueous solution of glutaraldehyde to the emulsion. The meeting and fusion of glutaraldehyde aqueous droplets with the ones containing the protein is a statistical phenomenon which is not easy to control. In the *modified procedure of Willmott* and co-workers, the glutaraldehyde solution is added to the aqueous protein solution just before emulsification [8; 111-114]. In another *modified procedure from Longo* and co-workers, glutaraldehyde is dissolved in an organic phase prior to its addition to the emulsion, in order to facilitate the diffusion of the cross-linking reagent through the organic phase, and to give a more accurate control on the reaction time [115]. In this modified procedure, the surfactant in the external phase is replaced by high concentrations of polymers, and the subsequent reaction with glutaraldehyde in this sterically-stabilized emulsion produces more hydrophilic microspheres than the classical method (figure 13) [115-117]. The resulting microspheres produced by any of these techniques are then separated from the reaction medium and washed successively with organic solvents and with aqueous solutions. Finally, residual aldehyde groups present on the particles can be quenched by adding amino compounds to the microspheres [115].

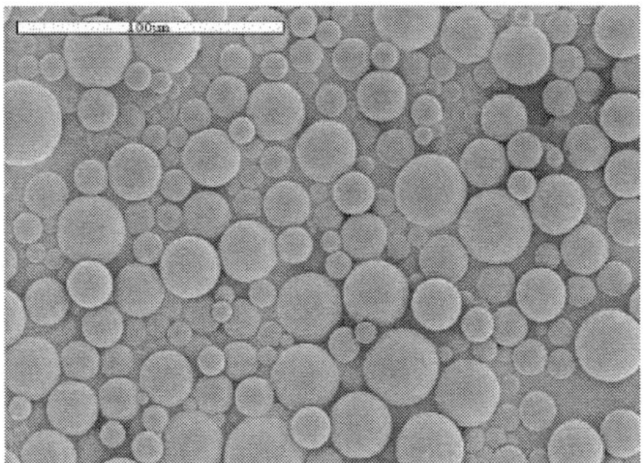

Figure 13. SEM microphotograph of mitoxantrone-loaded albumin microspheres prepared by the modified procedure of Longo (18). Reprinted from Almond BA et al., Journal of Controlled Release 2003; 91(1-2):147-155 with permission from Elsevier.

The size and size distribution of the microspheres is dependent on protein concentration, mixer design, stirring speed [118], proportion of oil in the emulsion [113], and when a monodisperse size distribution is desired, mostly if the particles are prepared for embolization, the procedure can include a sieving operation. Glutaraldehyde concentration influences size distribution too, but has also an effect on drug loading and release, and on enzymatic degradation of the particles [8; 119]. The addition of charged polyaminoacids to the initial protein solution can increase the particle content and slower the release of an inversely charged drug [111]. Comparing the release rate of progesterone from albumin microspheres prepared by different methods, the most rapid release was obtained from microspheres cross-linked with glutaraldehyde, as compared with microspheres prepared by the emulsification-thermal denaturation method [43].

Many studies deal with the use of the emulsification-cross-linking method for the encapsulation of drugs administered via various routes. Some of these studies are summarized in table 1. Another interesting application of glutaraldehyde-cross-linked microspheres has been studied by Shen and Mitragotri [30]. A novel drug delivery system consisting in albumin cross-linked microspheres embedded between two films has been proposed as an intestinal patch for oral drug delivery. This system includes a mucoadhesive permeable layer (carbopol-pectin film), a layer comprising drug-loaded microspheres for protection and controlled release of the drug, and an external impermeable layer constituted of an ethyl cellulose film.

Another technique using *glutaraldehyde cross-linking* of albumin involves a *spray-drying step* to produce the particles. In this method, explored by D'Souza and co-workers for more than ten years, the cross-linking step can be carried out after the spray-drying step, or the glutaraldehyde solution can be mixed to the albumin-drug solution just before atomization. This method has been applied to the encapsulation of many drugs to obtain a slow release of the drug [26; 125-128], a protection of the drug for oral administration [29; 129-131] or for another route [125; 126; 132], an increase of the cellular uptake of the drug [133; 134], and the diminution of side effects [134-136].

Table 1. Some studies on drug encapsulation in albumin microspheres prepared with the emulsion-cross-linking method

Encapsulated drug	Route of administration	Encapsulation aim	Reference
Doxorubicin	Intravenous	Embolization	[8; 111; 113; 114; 118]
Terbutaline sulfate	Intravenous	Passive lung targeting	[120]
Celecoxib	Intravenous	Inflammation targeting	[121]
Mitoxantrone	Intratumoral	Slow local release	[18]
Sodium naproxen	Intraarticular	Slow local release	[19]
Curcumin	Intraarticular	Slow local release	[96]
Hydralazine HCl	Intramuscular	Slow release	[122]
Ketorolac-tromethamine	Intramuscular	Slow release	[123]
Ketoprofen	Intramuscular	Slow release	[16]
Cytarabine	Subcutaneous implant in a film	Slow release	[22]
Iron	Oral	Increase uptake	[124]

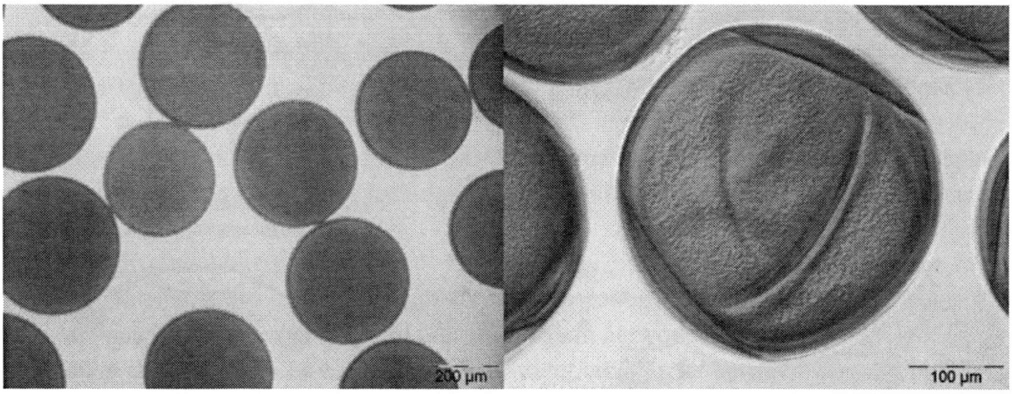

Figure 17. Optical microphotographs of serum albumin microcapsules cross-linked with TC, direct observation after staining with methylene blue (left), and detailed observation of the pleated membranes with interferential phase contrast [162].

Cross-linking of proteins can be achieved without cross-linking reagents, by activating a chemical group on the protein, which will react with another functional group, producing a *zero-length cross-linking* [107]. Microspheres for temporary arterial embolization have been produced in an emulsion system by zero-length cross-linking of human serum albumin [9]. The dispersed aqueous phase contained a mixture of albumin and carbodiimide for the activation of carboxyl groups of the protein and further reaction with amino groups to form *in situ* a network linked through amide bonds.

Another zero-length cross-linking method, which requires the presence of two biopolymers, is based on a *transacylation reaction* between a polysaccharidic ester, like propylene glycol alginate, and a protein. The carboxyl groups of the polysaccharide are activated in the form of esters, and the transacylation reaction, starting upon alkalization, produces amide bonds between the two biopolymers (figure 18). A thermostable gel is obtained, consisting of a covalent network produced in mild conditions without any toxic reactant.

The reaction has been adapted to microencapsulation by Edwards-Lévy and co-workers [163; 164]. Stable and biodegradable membranes with controllable thicknesses and interesting mechanical resistance could be created around hydrogel beads [163; 165-168](Figure 19). The membranes are formed of a hydrophilic network constituted of albumin directly bound to alginate through amide bonds, without any added cross-linking agent.

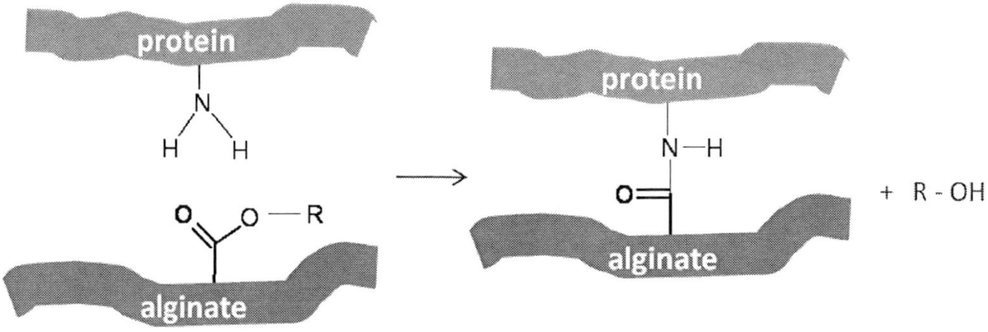

Figure 18. Transacylation reaction between a protein and an ester of alginic acid.

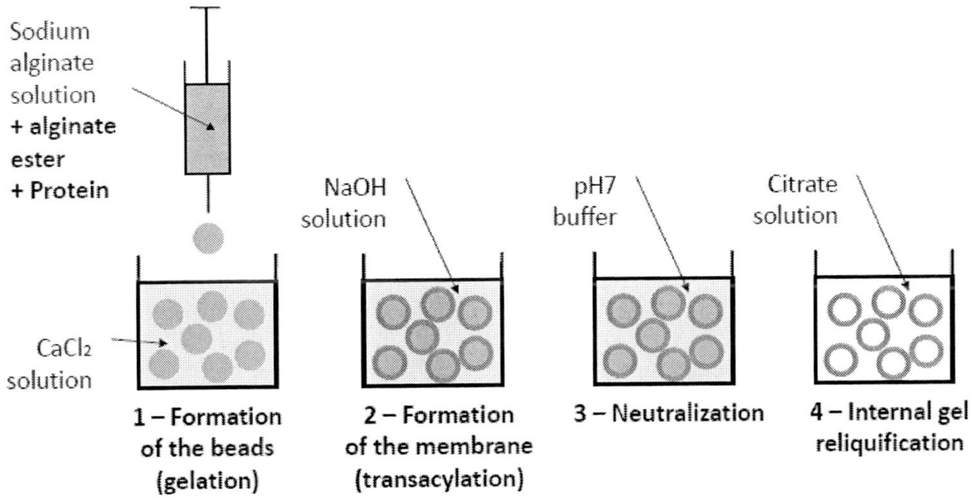

Figure 19. Preparation of membrane-coated calcium alginate beads using the transacylation reaction.

The particularly mild conditions required for the preparation of the capsules adapted very well to bioencapsulation (figure 20), and the covalent membrane showed a better stability as compared with the polyionic alginate-polylysine membrane classically used since the studies of Lim and Sun [169]. The encapsulation of several cell types showed a high preservation of cell viability and functionality [21; 170].

Calcium alginate microspheres were stabilized by encapsulation in a polysaccharide-protein covalent membrane and these particles were shown to release a bioactive peptide by an ion-exchange mechanism [20; 23; 24; 171].

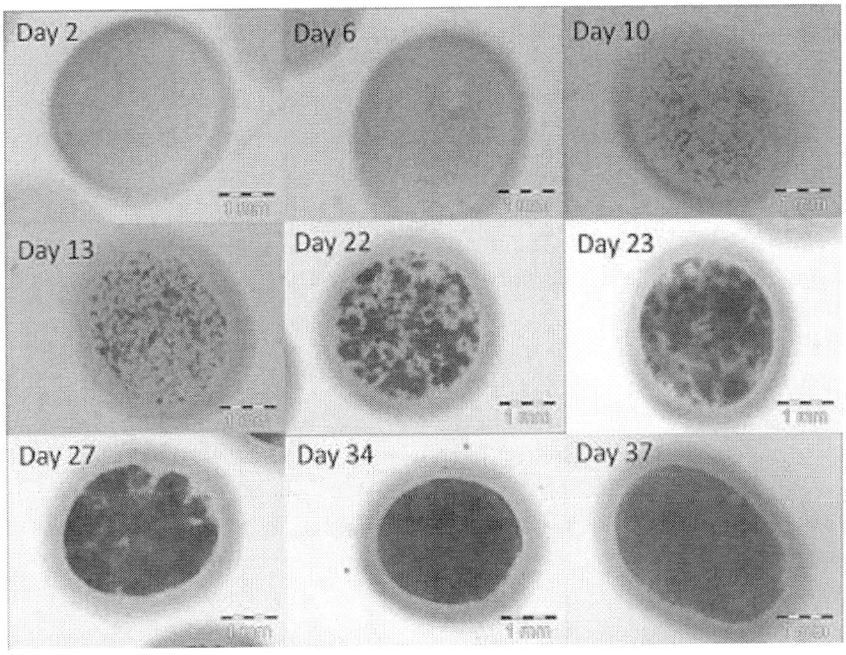

Figure 20. albumin-alginate coated beads containing the Jurkat cell line after various times in culture medium at 37°C [172].

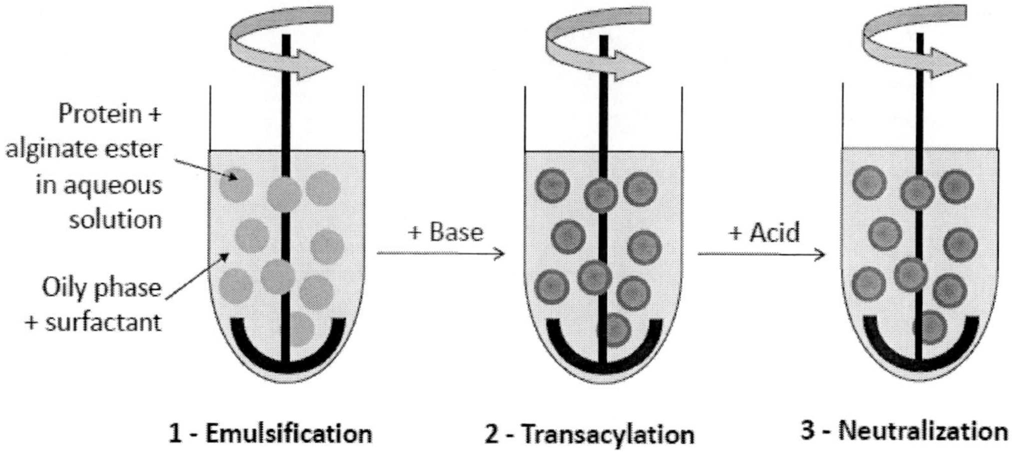

Figure 21. Preparation of albumin-alginate covalent microspheres by emulsion-transacylation.

Microparticles constituted of the polysaccharide-protein covalent network without calcium alginate gel have also been prepared, by starting the transacylation in an emulsion system where the dispersed aqueous phase contained the two biopolymers (figure 21) [20; 171]. This gentle procedure leads to stable, biocompatible and bio-degradable microparticles.

-Serum Albumin as an Additive in the Preparation of Microparticles

In the methods described above, serum albumin was involved in the network constituting the microparticles.

Many other studies use *albumin as a model protein* to study the release kinetics of proteins from microparticles, or to localize the protein in the microparticle structure. In most cases albumin is labeled with a fluorescent moiety such as fluorescein isothiocyanate, for visualization with a fluorescence microscope or for fluorimetric assay in a release medium [173]. Albumin can also serve as a model compound to study molecular imprinting onto microsphere surfaces [174], or to develop methods for protein grafting onto microspheres [175].

Due to the affinity of albumin for interfaces, this protein can in some cases advantageously replace *surfactants* in microencapsulation processes involving an emulsification step [176-180].

Serum albumin can also be incorporated as a *protective additive* in microparticles containing fragile biomolecules like growth factors [178], enzymes [181] or proteic hormones [182; 183], or in particles encapsulating living cells [21; 170; 184].

In vivo, serum albumin plays a role in controlling the osmotic pressure in the bloodstream. Lee and co-workers suggested the use of albumin as an *osmotic agent* to produce uniform open porous structures in polymer microspheres by inducing osmosis between internal and external phases during a double emulsion process [185]. The pores created by this technique presented a uniform size which was controlled by the albumin concentration, and the microsphere sizes were not affected by the presence of the porogen (figure 22).

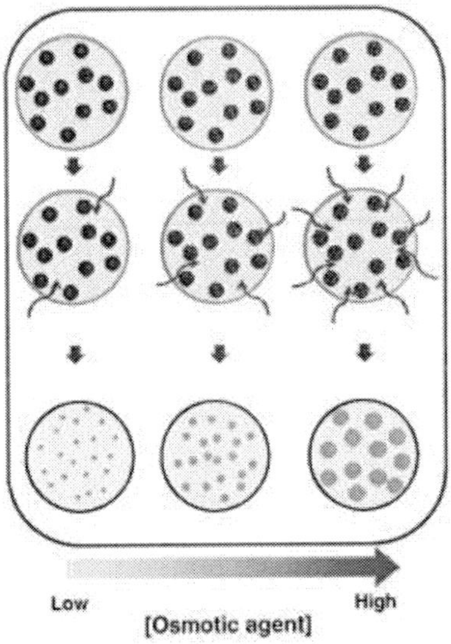

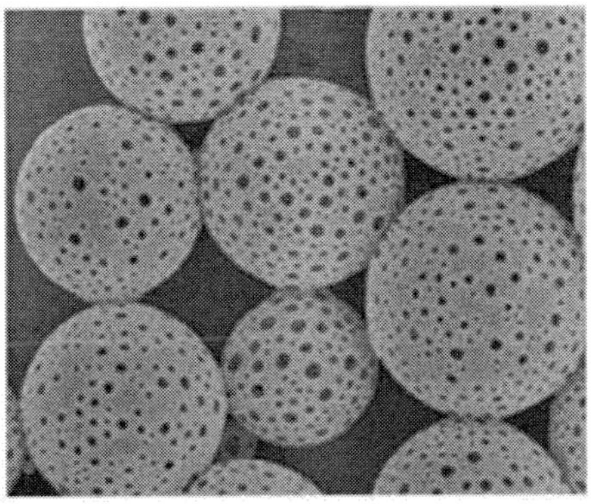

Figure 22. Preparation of microspheres of controlled pore size using albumin as a porogen (185). Reprinted from Lee J et al., Journal of Controlled Release 2010; 146(1):61-67 with permission from Elsevier.

- *Methods Involving Ovalbumin*

Some microencapsulation methods described or studied in the literature use egg white albumin instead of human or bovine serum albumin as membrane-forming or matrix-forming material. Although ovalbumin is not a pure protein and possesses slightly different physicochemical properties, the methods used to produce microparticles from ovalbumin can be easily transposed from those used for serum albumin. For example, the *emulsification-thermal denaturation* method has been applied to the preparation of ovalbumin microspheres containing pilocarpine [186] for ocular delivery. The *spray-drying method coupled with thermal denaturation* was used for the preparation of ovalbumin microparticles suitable for lung delivery [28]. Ovalbumin can also play the role of a *model compound* in the development of microspheres for molecular imprinting [187].

The *interfacial cross-linking* of ovalbumin with terephthaloyl chloride produced microcapsules which elastic properties were assessed by a novel method involving microfluidic technology [188]. The method consists in determining the deformation profiles of the microcapsules in microfluidic circuits and comparing the experimental deformation profiles with theoretical profiles obtained from mathematical modeling. The values obtained with microcapsules prepared varying the cross-linking reaction conditions correlated well with the values of cross-linking degrees of the membranes obtained from a chemical assay [189].

The precipitation of albumin from its aqueous solution divided in droplets in an emulsion system can be started upon *addition of lactic acid under moderate heating* [190]. The particles obtained by lactic acid precipitation presented a better stability than the heated only particles. This means of ovalbumin stabilization, although the mechanism is not elucidated yet, is promising, as lactic acid is a biocompatible endogeneous compound.

CONCLUSION

Among the different drug delivery systems, microparticles offer unique features for the improvement of efficacy of drugs. Serum albumin presents interesting properties for its use as a raw material in microparticle preparation.

However, serum albumin microparticles available for applications in health are not numerous. Albumin microbubbles (Albunex® from Mallinckrodt Inc., Optison® from GE Healthcare Medical Diagnostics) are being used as echo contrast agents in clinical ultrasound imaging, and heat-denaturated albumin microspheres (Rotop Pharmaka AG, Germany) are useful for lung perfusion imaging after labeling with ^{99m}Tc. The other available microparticles are constituted of synthetic or semi-synthetic polymers.

The literature offers a large panel of studies dealing with the development of encapsulation methods using serum albumin. Their applications to the delivery of various drugs by different routes are being studied. The novel methods offer a better safety for health applications, and the parameters leading to the desired properties are controlled. Furthermore, the recent marketing of Abraxane®, containing albumin nanoparticles loaded with paclitaxel, certainly opens the way for other particulate systems based on albumin.

ACKNOWLEDGMENTS

Quentin Ribour is gratefully acknowledged for the assistance in drawing some of the figures.

REFERENCES

[1] Patil GV. Biopolymer albumin for diagnosis and in drug delivery. *Drug Development Research* 2003; 58(3):219-247.

[2] Kratz F. Albumin as a drug carrier: Design of prodrugs, drug conjugates and nanoparticles. *Journal of Controlled Release* 2008; 132(3):171-183.

[3] Arshady R. Microspheres Microcapsules and Liposomes: Preparation and chemical applications. *Citus Books*; 1999.

[4] Benita S. Microencapsulation: methods and industrial applications. Taylor and Francis; 2006.

[5] Shanthi CN, Gupta R, *Mahato AK. Traditional and emerging applications of microspheres: A review. International Journal of PharmTech Research* 2010; 2(1):675-681.

[6] Banquet S, Gomez E, Nicol L, Edwards-Lévy F, Henry J-P, Cao R, Schapman D, Dautreaux B, Lallemand F, Bauer F, Cao Y, Richard V, Mulder P, Thuillez C, Brakenhielm E. Arteriogenic therapy by intramyocardial sustained delivery of a novel growth factor combination prevents chronic heart failure. Circulation, in press.

[7] Kouchakzadeh H, Shojaosadati SA, Maghsoudi A, Vasheghani Farahani E. Optimization of PEGylation conditions for BSA nanoparticles using response surface methodology. *AAPS PharmSciTech* 2010; 11(3):1206-1211.

[8] Willmott N, Cummings J, Stuart JFB, Florence AT. Adriamycin-loaded albumin microspheres: Preparation, in vivo distribution and release in the rat. *Biopharmaceutics and Drug Disposition* 1985; 6(1):91-104.
[9] Schwarz A, Zhang H, Metcalfe A, Salazkin I, Raymond J. Transcatheter embolization using degradable crosslinked hydrogels. *Biomaterials* 2004; 25(21):5209-5215.
[10] Benita S, Fickat R, Benoît JP, Bonnemain B, Samaille JP, Madoulé P. Biodegradable cross-linked albumin microcapsules for embolization. *Journal of Microencapsulation* 1984; 1(4):317-327.
[11] Nijsen JFW, van het Schip AD, Hennink WE, Rook DW, van Rijk PP, de Klerk JMH. Advances in nuclear oncology: Microspheres for internal radionuclide therapy in liver tumours. *Current Medicinal Chemistry* 2002; 9(1):73-82.
[12] Toublan FJ-J, Boppart S, Suslick KS. Tumor targeting by surface-modified protein microspheres. *Journal of the American Chemical Society* 2006; 128(11):3472-3473.
[13] Lawrie A, Brisken AF, Francis SE, Cumberland DC, Crossman DC, Newman CM. Microbubble-enhanced ultrasound for vascular gene delivery. *Gene Therapy* 2000; 7(23):2023-2027.
[14] Takeuchi H, Ohmori K, Kondo I, Shinomiya K, Oshita A, Takagi Y, Yoshida J, Mizushige K, Kohno M. Interaction with Leukocytes: Phospholipid-stabilized versus Albumin-Shell Microbubbles. *Radiology* 2004; 230(3):735-742.
[15] Brusentsov NA, Baiburtskii FS, Tarasov VV, Komissarova LK, Filippov VI. Production technology and application of polyfunctional magnetically guided superparamagnetic preparations (a review). *Pharmaceutical Chemistry Journal* 2002; 36(4):197-205.
[16] Mathew ST, Gayathri Devi S, Prasanth VV, Vinod B. Formulation and in vitroin vivo evaluation of ketoprofen-loaded albumin microspheres for intramuscular administration. *Journal of Microencapsulation* 2009; 26(5):456-469.
[17] Eatock M, Church N, Harris R, Angerson W, McArdle C, French R, Twelves C. Activity of doxorubicin covalently bound to a novel human serum albumin microcapsule. *Investigational New Drugs* 1999; 17(2):111-120.
[18] Almond BA, Hadba AR, Freeman ST, Cuevas BJ, York AM, Detrisac CJ, Goldberg EP. Efficacy of mitoxantrone-loaded albumin microspheres for intratumoral chemotherapy of breast cancer. *Journal of Controlled Release* 2003; 91(1-2):147-155.
[19] Bozdağ S, Çaliş S, Kaş HS, Ercan MT, Peksoy I, Hincal AA. In vitro evaluation and intra-articular administration of biodegradable microspheres containing naproxen sodium. *Journal of Microencapsulation* 2001; 18(4):443-456.
[20] Callewaert M, Millot J-M, Lesage J, Laurent-Maquin D, Edwards-Lévy F. Serum albumin-alginate coated microspheres: Role of the inner gel in binding and release of the KRFK peptide. *International Journal of Pharmaceutics* 2009; 366(1-2):103-110.
[21] Shinya E, Dervillez X, Edwards-Lévy F, Duret V, Brisson E, Ylisastigui L, Lévy MC, Cohen JHM, Klatzmann D. In-vivo delivery of therapeutic proteins by genetically-modified cells: Comparison of organoids and human serum albumin alginate-coated beads. *Biomedicine and Pharmacotherapy* 1999; 53(10):471-483.
[22] Gómez C, Blanco MD, Bernardo MV, Olmo R, Muñiz E, Teijón JM. Cytarabine release from comatrices of albumin microspheres in a poly(lactide-co-glycolide) film: In vitro and in vivo studies. *European Journal of Pharmaceutics and Biopharmaceutics* 2004; 57(2):225-233.

[23] Hurteaux R, Benhayoune H, Edwards-Levy F, Bouthors S, Balossier G, Laurent-Maquin D. Preparation and characterization of an electrodeposited calcium phosphate coating associated with a calcium alginate matrix. *Journal of Materials Science: Materials in Medicine* 2005; 16(1):9-13.

[24] Hurteaux R, Edwards-Lévy F, Laurent-Maquin D, Lévy M-C. Coating alginate microspheres with a serum albumin-alginate membrane: Application to the encapsulation of a peptide. *European Journal of Pharmaceutical Sciences* 2005; 24(2-3):187-197.

[25] Pereswetoff-Morath L. Microspheres as nasal drug delivery systems. *Advanced Drug Delivery Reviews* 1998; 29(1-2):185-194.

[26] Addo RT, Siddig A, Siwale R, Patel NJ, Akande J, Uddin AN, D'Souza MJ. Formulation, characterization and testing of tetracaine hydrochloride-loaded albumin-chitosan microparticles for ocular drug delivery. *Journal of Microencapsulation* 2010; 27(2):95-104.

[27] Della Porta G, Adami R, Del Gaudio P, Prota L, Aquino R, Reverchon E. Albumin/gentamicin microspheres produced by supercritical assisted atomization: Optimization of size, drug loading and release. *Journal of Pharmaceutical Sciences* 2010; 99(11):4720-4729.

[28] Sivadas N, O'Rourke D, Tobin A, Buckley V, Ramtoola Z, Kelly JG, Hickey AJ, Cryan S-A. A comparative study of a range of polymeric microspheres as potential carriers for the inhalation of proteins. *International Journal of Pharmaceutics* 2008; 358(1-2): 159-167.

[29] Lanke SSS, Gayakwad SG, Strom JG, D'Souza MJ. Oral delivery of low molecular weight heparin microspheres prepared using biodegradable polymer matrix system. *Journal of Microencapsulation* 2009; 26(6):493-500.

[30] Shen Z, Mitragotri S. Intestinal patches for oral drug delivery. *Pharmaceutical Research* 2002; 19(4):391-395.

[31] Reverchon E, Antonacci A. Drug-polymer microparticles produced by supercritical assisted atomization. *Biotechnology and Bioengineering* 2007; 97(6): 1626-1637.

[32] Chatterjee J, Haik Y, Chen C-J. Synthesis and characterization of heat-stabilized albumin magnetic microspheres. *Colloid and Polymer Science* 2001; 279(11): 1073-1081.

[33] Muramatsu N, Kondo T. An approach to prepare microparticles of uniform size. *Journal of Microencapsulation* 1995; 12(2):129-136.

[34] Chen C-Y, Long Q, Li X-H, Xu J. Microwave-assisted preparation of magnetic albumin microspheres. *Journal of Bioactive and Compatible Polymers* 2008; 23(5): 490-500.

[35] Kramer PA, Burnstein T. Phagocytosis of microspheres containing an anticancer agent by tumor cells in vitro. *Life Sciences* 1976; 19(4):515-519.

[36] Kramer PA. Albumin microspheres as vehicles for achieving specificity in drug delivery. *Journal of Pharmaceutical Sciences* 1974; 63(10):1646-1647.

[37] Sugibayashi K, Akimoto M, Morimoto Y. Drug-carrier property of albumin microspheres in chemotherapy. III. Effect of microsphere-entrapped 5-fluorouracil on Ehrlich ascites carcinoma in mice. *Journal of Pharmacobio-Dynamics* 1979; 2(6): 350-355.

[38] Morimoto Y, Akimoto M, Sugibayashi K. Drug-carrier property of albumin microspheres in chemotherapy. IV. Antitumor effect of single-shot or multiple-shot administration of microsphere-entrapped 5-fluorouracil on Ehrlich ascites or solid tumor in mice. *Chemical and Pharmaceutical Bulletin* 1980; 28(10):3087-3092.
[39] Jia WJ, Liu JG, De Zhang Y, Wang JW, Wang J, Sun CY, Pan YF, Yu C, Li GZ, Zhang H, Gou ML, Tu MJ, Qian ZY. Preparation, characterization, and optimization of pancreas-targeted 5-Fu loaded magnetic bovine serum albumin microspheres. *Journal of Drug Targeting* 2007; 15(2):140-145.
[40] Tian Y, Klegerman ME, Hickey AJ. Evaluation of microparticles containing doxorubicin suitable for aerosol delivery to the lungs. *PDA Journal of Pharmaceutical Science and Technol*ogy 2004; 58(5):266-275.
[41] Sarojini S, Prem Kumar A, Pradeep D, Manavalan R, Jayanthi B. Formulation and evaluation of albumin-chitosan floating microsphere containing clarithromycin and estimation by spectrophotometric method. *Research Journal of Pharmaceutical, Biological and Chemical Sciences* 2010; 1(2):207-214.
[42] Orienti I. Influence of physico-chemical parameters on the release of hydrocortisone acetate from albumin microspheres. *Journal of Controlled Release* 1994; 31(1):61-71.
[43] Orienti I, Zecchi V. Progesterone-loaded albumin microparticles. *Journal of Controlled Release* 1993; 27(1):1-7.
[44] Vyas SP, Bhatnagar S, Gogoi PJ, Jain NK. Preparation and characterization of HSA-propranolol microspheres for nasal administration. *International Journal of Pharmaceutics* 1991; 69(1):5-12.
[45] European Pharmacopoeia. 7th ed. EDQM; 2011.
[46] Zolle I. Technetium-99m pharmaceuticals: preparation and quality control in nuclear medicine. Springer; 2007.
[47] Vente MAD, Zonnenberg BA, Nijsen JFW. Microspheres for radioembolization of liver malignancies. *Expert Review of Medical Devices* 2010; 7(5):581-583.
[48] Chuang VTG, Kragh-Hansen U, Otagiri M. Pharmaceutical strategies utilizing recombinant human serum albumin. *Pharmaceutical Research* 2002; 19(5):569-577.
[49] Perkins AC, Frier M. Experimental biodistribution studies of 99mTc-recombinant human serum albumin (rHSA): A new generation of radiopharmaceutical. *European Journal of Nuclear Medicine* 1994; 21(11):1231-1233.
[50] Pasqualini R, Plassio G, Sosi S. The preparation of albumin microspheres. *The Journal of nuclear biology and medicine* 1969; 13(1):80-84.
[51] Ahmadzadehfar H, Sabet A, Muckle M, Wilhelm K, Reichmann K, Biersack H-J, Ezziddin S. 99mTc-MAA/90Y-Bremsstrahlung SPECT/CT after simultaneous Tc-MAA/90Y-microsphere injection for immediate treatment monitoring and further therapy planning for radioembolization. *European Journal of Nuclear Medicine and Molecular Imaging* 2011; 38(7):1281-1288.
[52] Schiller E, Bergmann R, Pietzsch J, Noll B, Sterger A, Johannsen B, Wunderlich G, Pietzsch H-J. Yttrium-86-labelled human serum albumin microspheres: relation of surface structure with in vivo stability. *Nuclear Medicine and Biology* 2008; 35(2):227-232.
[53] Wunderlich G, Drews A, Kotzerke J. A kit for labeling of [188Re] human serum albumin microspheres for therapeutic use in nuclear medicine. *Applied Radiation and Isotopes* 2005; 62(6):915-918.

[54] Wunderlich G, Schiller E, Bergmann R, Pietzsch H-J. Comparison of the stability of Y-90-, Lu-177- and Ga-68- labeled human serum albumin microspheres (DOTA-HSAM). *Nuclear Medicine and Biology* 2010; 37(8):861-867.

[55] Borza VN, Neacsu E, Barna CM, Popescu-Pogrion N, Mercioniu L, Nistor CL. Labelling of albumin microspheres with 188Re: A possible agent for radiotherapy. *International Journal of Nano and Biomaterials* 2009; 2(6):540-546.

[56] Borza VN, Neacsu E, Mustaciosu C, Luca A, Barna C, Popescu N, Mercioniu I, Albert P, Hurduc A, Moldovan L, Savi GP, Savi I, Matei L. Rhenium-188 labelled albumin microspheres for therapy of liver tumors. *Journal of Labelled Compounds and Radiopharmaceuticals* 2010; 53(5-6):470-471.

[57] McDonald MA, Watkin KL. Small particulate gadolinium oxide and gadolinium oxide albumin microspheres as multimodal contrast and therapeutic agents. *Investigative Radiology* 2003; 38(6):305-310.

[58] Wang J, Wang X, Ren L, Wang Q, Li L, Liu W, Wan Z, Yang L, Sun P, Ren L, Li M, Wu H, Wang J, Zhang L. Conjugation of biomolecules with magnetic protein microspheres for the assay of early biomarkers associated with acute myocardial infarction. *Analytical Chemistry* 2009; 81(15):6210-6217.

[59] Widder KJ, Morris RM, Poore G. Tumor remission in Yoshida sarcoma-bearing rats by selective targeting of magnetic albumin microspheres containing doxorubicin. Proceedings of the National Academy of Sciences of the United States of America 1981; 78(1 II):579-581.

[60] Widder K, Flouret G, Senyei A. Magnetic microspheres: synthesis of a novel parenteral drug carrier. *Journal of Pharmaceutical Sciences* 1979; 68(1):79-82.

[61] Widder KJ, Senyei AE, Scarpelli DG. Magnetic microspheres: A model system for site specific drug delivery in vivo. *Proceedings of the Society for Experimental Biology and Medicine* 1978; 158(2):141-146.

[62] Giunchedi P, Conte U. Spray-drying as a preparation method of microparticulate drug delivery systems: An overview. S.T.P. Pharma Pratiques 1995; 5(4):276-290.

[63] Maa Y-F, Costantino HR, Nguyen P-A, Hsu CC. The effect of operating and formulation variables on the morphology of spray-dried protein particles. *Pharmaceutical Development and Technology* 1997; 2(3):213-223.

[64] Vehring R. Pharmaceutical particle engineering via spray drying. *Pharmaceutical Research* 2008; 25(5):999-1022.

[65] Li FQ, Hu JH, Lu B, Yao H, Zhang WG. Ciprofloxacin-loaded bovine serum albumin microspheres: Preparation and drug-release in vitro. *Journal of Microencapsulation* 2001; 18(6):825-829.

[66] Conte U, Giunchedi P, Maggi L, Torre ML. Spray dried albumin microspheres containing nicardipine. *European Journal of Pharmaceutics and Biopharmaceutics* 1994; 40(4):203-208.

[67] Sánchez-Brunete JA, Dea MA, Rama S, Bolás F, Alunda JM, Raposo R, Méndez MT, Torrado-Santiago S, Torrado JJ. Treatment of experimental visceral leishmaniasis with amphotericin B in stable albumin microspheres. *Antimicrobial Agents and Chemotherapy* 2004; 48(9):3246-3252.

[68] Das S, Khan W, Mohsin S, Kumar N. Miltefosine loaded albumin microparticles for treatment of visceral leishmaniasis: Formulation development and in vitro evaluation. *Polymers for Advanced Technologies* 2011; 22(1):172-179.

[69] Khan W, Kumar N. Drug targeting to macrophages using paromomycin-loaded albumin microspheres for treatment of visceral leishmaniasis: An in vitro evaluation. *Journal of Drug Targeting* 2011; 19(4):239-250.

[70] Chu M, Zhou L, Song X, Pan M, Zhang L, Sun Y, Zhu J, Ding Z. Incorporating quantum dots into polymer microspheres via a spray-drying and thermal-denaturizing approach. *Nanotechnology* 2006; 17(6):1791-1796.

[71] Wang Q, Guan Y-X, Yao S-J, Zhu Z-Q. Controllable preparation and formation mechanism of BSA microparticles using supercritical assisted atomization with an enhanced mixer. *Journal of Supercritical Fluids* 2011; 56(1):97-104.

[72] Yu Z, Garcia AS, Johnston KP, Williams III RO. Spray freezing into liquid nitrogen for highly stable protein nanostructured microparticles. *European Journal of Pharmaceutics and Biopharmaceutics* 2004; 58(3):529-537.

[73] Gedanken A. Preparation and properties of proteinaceous microspheres made sonochemically. *Chemistry - A European Journal* 2008; 14(13):3840-3853.

[74] Grinstaff MW, Suslick KS. Protein microencapsulation of nonaqueous liquids. *Journal of the American Chemical Society* 1990; 112:7807-7809.

[75] Grinstaff MW, Suslick KS. Nonaqueous liquid filled microcapsules. American Chemical Society, *Polymer Preprints*, *Division of Polymer Chemistry* 1991; 32: 255-256.

[76] Suslick KS, Grinstaff MW, Kolbeck KJ, Wong M. Characterization of sonochemically prepared proteinaceous microspheres. *Ultrasonics - Sonochemistry* 1994; 1(1):S65-S68.

[77] Avivi S, Gedanken A. S-S bonds are not required for the sonochemical formation of proteinaceous microspheres: The case of streptavidin. *Biochemical Journal* 2002; 366(3):705-707.

[78] Makino K, Mizorogi T, Ando S, Tsukamoto T, Ohshima H. Sonochemically prepared bovine serum albumin microcapsules: Factors affecting the size distribution and the microencapsulation yield. *Colloids and Surfaces B*: *Biointerfaces* 2001; 22(3):251-255.

[79] Makino K, Mizorogi T, Ando S, Tsukamoto T, Ohshima H. Sustained release of hydrophobic materials from sonochemically prepared bovine serum albumin microcapsules. *Colloids and Surfaces B: Biointerfaces* 2002; 23(1):59-64.

[80] Angel U, Matas D, Michaeli S, Cavaco-Paulo A, Gedanken A. Microspheres of mixed proteins. *Chemistry - A European Journal* 2010; 16(7):2108-2114.

[81] Grinberg O, Gedanken A, Patra CR, Patra S, Mukherjee P, Mukhopadhyay D. Sonochemically prepared BSA microspheres containing Gemcitabine, and their potential application in renal cancer therapeutics. *Acta Biomaterialia* 2009; 5(8): 3031-3037.

[82] Grinberg O, Hayun M, Sredni B, Gedanken A. Characterization and activity of sonochemically-prepared BSA microspheres containing Taxol - An anticancer drug. *Ultrasonics Sonochemistry* 2007; 14(5):661-666.

[83] Avivi S, Nitzan Y, Dror R, Gedanken A. An Easy Sonochemical Route for the Encapsulation of Tetracycline in Bovine Serum Albumin Microspheres. *Journal of the American Chemical Socie*ty 2003; 125(51):15712-15713.

[84] Avivi S, Felner I, Novik I, Gedanken A. The preparation of magnetic proteinaceous microspheres using the sonochemical method. *Biochimica et Biophysica Acta - General Subjects* 2001; 1527(3):123-129.

[85] Jiang W, Sun Z, Li F, Chen K, Liu T, Liu J, Zhou T, Guo R. A novel approach to preparing magnetic protein microspheres with core-shell structure. *Journal of Magnetism and Magnetic Materials* 2011; 323(5):435-439.
[86] Langer K, Anhorn MG, Steinhauser I, Dreis S, Celebi D, Schrickel N, Faust S, Vogel V. Human serum albumin (HSA) nanoparticles: Reproducibility of preparation process and kinetics of enzymatic degradation. *International Journal of Pharmaceutics* 2008; 347(1-2):109-117.
[87] Langer K, Balthasar S, Vogel V, Dinauer N, Von Briesen H, Schubert D. Optimization of the preparation process for human serum albumin (HSA) nanoparticles. *International Journal of Pharmaceutics* 2003; 257(1-2):169-180.
[88] Weber C, Kreuter J, Langer K. Desolvation process and surface characteristics of HSA-nanoparticles. *International Journal of Pharmaceutics* 2000; 196(2):197-200.
[89] Zhu Y, Tong W, Gao C, Möhwald H. Fabrication of bovine serum albumin microcapsules by desolvation and destroyable cross-linking. *Journal of Materials Chemistry* 2008; 18(10):1153-1158.
[90] De Kruif CG, Weinbreck F, De Vries R. Complex coacervation of proteins and anionic polysaccharides. *Current Opinion in Colloid and Interface Science* 2004; 9(5):340-349.
[91] Green BK, Schleicher L, The National Cash Register Company. Oil-Containing Microscopic Capsules and Method of Making Them. US patent 1957; 2 800 457
[92] Singh ON, Burgess DJ. Characterization of albumin-alginic acid complex coacervation. *Journal of Pharmacy and Pharmacology* 1989; 41(10):670-673.
[93] Burgess NJ, Singh NO. Spontaneous formation of small sized albumin/acacia coacervate particles. *Journal of Pharmacy and Pharmacology* 1993; 45(7):586-591.
[94] Galazka VB, Ledward DA, Sumner IG, Dickinson E. Influence of High Pressure on Bovine Serum Albumin and Its Complex with Dextran Sulfate. *Journal of Agricultural and Food Chemistry* 1997; 45(9):3465-3471.
[95] Galazka VB, Smith D, Ledward DA, Dickinson E. Complexes of bovine serum albumin with sulphated polysaccharides: Effects of pH, ionic strength and high pressure treatment. *Food Chemistry* 1999; 64(3):303-310.
[96] Kumar V, Lewis SA, Mutalik S, Shenoy DB, Venkatesh, Udupa N. Biodegradable microspheres of curcumin for treatment of inflammation. *Indian Journal of Physiology and Pharmacology* 2002; 46(2):209-217.
[97] Lu G, An Z, Tao C, Li J. Microcapsule assembly of human serum albumin at the liquid/liquid interface by the pendent drop technique. *Langmuir* 2004; 20(19): 8401-8403.
[98] Lvov Y, Ariga K, Ichinose I, Kunitake T. Assembly of multicomponent protein films by means of electrostatic layer-by-layer adsorption. *Journal of the American Chemical Society* 1995; 117(22):6117-6123.
[99] De Cock LJ, De Koker S, De Geest BG, Grooten J, Vervaet C, Remon JP, Sukhorukov GB, Antipina MN. Polymeric Multilayer Capsules in Drug Delivery. *Angewandte Chemie - International Edition* 2010; 49(39):6954-6973.
[100] Peyratout CS, Dähne L. Tailor-made polyelectrolyte microcapsules: From multilayers to smart containers. *Angewandte Chemie - International Edition* 2004; 43(29): 3762-3783.

[101] An Z, Lu G, Möhwald H, Li J. Self-assembly of human serum albumin (HSA) and L-α-dimyristoylphosphatidic acid (DMPA) microcapsules for controlled drug release. *Chemistry - A European Journal* 2004; 10(22):5848-5852.
[102] An Z, Möhwald H, Li J. pH controlled permeability of lipid/protein biomimetic microcapsules. *Biomacromolecules* 2006; 7(2):580-585.
[103] An Z, Tao C, Lu G, Möhwald H, Zheng S, Cui Y, Li J. Fabrication and characterization of human serum albumin and L-α-dimyristoylphosphatidic acid microcapsules based on template technique. *Chemistry of Materials* 2005; 17(10):2514-2519.
[104] Balkundi SS, Veerabadran NG, Matthew Eby D, Johnson GR, Lvov YM. Encapsulation of bacterial spores in nanoorganized polyelectrolyte shells. *Langmuir* 2009; 25(24):14011-14016.
[105] Lu G, An Z, Li J. Biogenic capsules made of proteins and lipids. *Biochemical and Biophysical Research Communications* 2004; 315(1):224-227.
[106] Tong W, Gao C, Möhwald H. pH-responsive protein microcapsules fabricated via glutaraldehyde mediated covalent layer-by-layer assembly. *Colloid and Polymer Science* 2008; 286(10):1103-1109.
[107] Wong SS. Chemistry of protein conjugation and cross-linking. CRC Press; 1993.
[108] Katti D, Krishnamurti N. Preparation of albumin microspheres by an improved process. *Journal of Microencapsulation* 1999; 16(2):231-242.
[109] Wang C, Liu J, Gao Q, Bi Y, Gan L, Wang X, Hou S. Preparation and characterization of Pingyangmycin-loaded bovine serum albumin microspheres for embolization therapy. *International Journal of Pharmaceutics* 2007; 336(2):361-366.
[110] Lee TK, Sokoloski TD, Royer GP. Serum albumin beads: An injectable, biodegradable system for the sustained release of drugs. *Science* 1981; 213(4504):233-235.
[111] Willmott N, Chen Y, Florence AT. Haemoglobin, transferrin and albumin/polyaspartic acid microspheres as carriers for the cytotoxic drug adriamycin. II. In vitro drug release rate. *Journal of Controlled Release* 1988; 8(2):103-109.
[112] Willmott N, Chen Y, Goldberg J, Mcardle C, Florence AT. Biodegradation rate of embolized protein microspheres in lung, liver and kidney of rats. *Journal of Pharmacy and Pharmacology* 1989; 41(7):433-438.
[113] Willmott N, Kamel HMH, Cummings J, Stuart JFB, Florence AT. Adriamycin-loaded albumin microspheres: Lung entrapment and fate in the rat. In: Microspheres and Drug Therapy. Pharmaceutical, Immunological and Medical Aspects. S.S. Davis, L. Illum, J.G. McVie and E. Tomlinson; 1984 p. 205-215.
[114] Cummings J, Willmott N. Adriamycin-loaded albumin microspheres: qualitative assessment of drug incorporation and in vitro release by high-performance liquid chromatography and high-speed multi-diode array spectrophotometric detection. *Journal of Chromatography Biomedical Applications* 1985; 343:208-212.
[115] Longo WE, Iwata H, Lindheimer TA, Goldberg EP. Preparation of hydrophilic albumin microspheres using polymeric dispersing agents. *Journal of Pharmaceutical Sciences* 1982; 71(12):1323-1328.
[116] Latha MS, Jayakrishnan A. A new method for the synthesis of smooth, round, hydrophilic protein microspheres using low concentrations of polymeric dispersing agents. *Journal of Microencapsulation* 1995; 12(1):7-12.

[117] Yan C, Kitano H, Ise N. Functional properties of proteins immobilized on albumin microspheres. *Biotechnol. Appl. Biochem.* 1988; 10:13-20.

[118] Tomlinson E, Burger JJ, Schoonderwoerd EMA. Preparation and characterisation of albumin microspheres for intraarterial tumour targetting of cytotoxic compounds. *Journal of Pharmacy and Pharmacology* 1982; 34(Suppl.):88P.

[119] Sheu M-T, Moustafa MA, Sokoloski TD. Entrapment of bioactive compounds within native albumin beads: II. Effects of rate and extent of crosslinking on microbead properties. *Journal of Parenteral Science and Technology* 1986; 40(6):253-258.

[120] Sahin S, Selek H, Ponchel G, Ercan MT, Sargon M, Hincal AA, Kas HS. Preparation, characterization and in vivo distribution of terbutaline sulfate loaded albumin microspheres. *Journal of Controlled Release* 2002; 82(2-3):345-358.

[121] Thakkar H, Sharma RK, Mishra AK, Chuttani K, Murthy RR. Albumin microspheres as carriers for the antiarthritic drug celecoxib. *AAPS PharmSciTech* 2005; 6(1):E65-E73.

[122] Nanjwade BK, Bechra HM, Nanjwade VK, Derkar GK, Manvi FV. Formulation and characterization of hydralazine hydrochloride biodegraded microspheres for intramuscular administration. *Journal of Bioanalysis and Biomedicine* 2011; 3(1): 32-37.

[123] Mathew ST, Devi SG, Sandhya KV. Formulation and evaluation of ketorolac tromethamine-loaded albumin microspheres for potential intramuscular administration. *AAPS PharmSciTech* 2007; 8(1)

[124] Shivakumar HN, Vaka SRK, Murthy SN. Albumin microspheres for oral delivery of iron. *Journal of Drug Targeting* 2010; 18(1):36-44.

[125] Okoroukwu ON, Green GR, D'Souza MJ. Development of albumin microspheres containing Sp H1-DNA complexes: A novel gene delivery system. *Journal of Microencapsulation* 2010; 27(2):142-149.

[126] Gayakwad SG, Bejugam NK, Akhavein N, Uddin NA, Oettinger CE, D'Souza MJ. Formulation and in vitro characterization of spray-dried antisense oligonucleotide to NF-B encapsulated albumin microspheres. *Journal of Microencapsulation* 2009; 26(8):692-700.

[127] Haswani DK, Nettey H, Oettinger C, D'Souza M. Formulation, characterization and pharmacokinetic evaluation of gentamicin sulphate loaded albumin microspheres. *Journal of Microencapsulation* 2006; 23(8):875-886.

[128] Nettey H, Haswani D, Oettinger CW, D'Souza MJ. Formulation and testing of vancomycin loaded albumin microspheres prepared by spray-drying. *Journal of Microencapsulation* 2006; 23(6):632-642.

[129] Yeboah KG, D'Souza MJ. Evaluation of albumin microspheres as oral delivery system for Mycobacterium tuberculosis vaccines. *Journal of Microencapsulation* 2009; 26(2):166-179.

[130] Uddin AN, Bejugam NK, Gayakwad SG, Akther P, D'Souza MJ. Oral delivery of gastro-resistant microencapsulated typhoid vaccine. *Journal of Drug Targeting* 2009; 17(7):553-560.

[131] Bejugam NK, Uddin AN, Gayakwad SG, D'Souza MJ. Formulation and evaluation of albumin microspheres and its enteric coating using a spray-dryer. *Journal of Microencapsulation* 2008; 25(8):577-583.

[132] Siwale RC, Oettinger CW, Balakrishna Pai S, Addo R, Uddin N, Siddig A, D'Souza MJ. Formulation and characterization of catalase in albumin microspheres. *Journal of Microencapsulation* 2009; 26(5):411-419.
[133] Haswani DK, Nettey H, D'Souza MJ, Oettinger CW. In vitro evaluation and targeting of E. coli internalized by endothelial cells using albumin microspheres loaded with gentamicin. *Drug Development and Industrial Pharmacy* 2007; 33(2):181-190.
[134] Do DP, Pai SB, Rizvi SAA, D'Souza MJ. Development of sulforaphane-encapsulated microspheres for cancer epigenetic therapy. *International Journal of Pharmaceutics* 2010; 386(1-2):114-121.
[135] Angra PK, Oettinger C, Balakrishna Pai S, D'Souza MJ. Amphotericin B microspheres: A therapeutic approach to minimize toxicity while maintaining antifungal efficacy. *Journal of Microencapsulation* 2009; 26(7):580-587.
[136] Angra PK, Siddig A, Nettey H, Desai N, Oettinger C, D'Souza MJ. Pharmacokinetic and biodistribution studies of Amphotericin B microspheres. *Journal of Microencapsulation* 2009; 26(7):627-634.
[137] Tao C, Chen D, Zhang J. The fabrication of hollow BSA micro/nanocapsules. *Journal of Nanoscience and Nanotechnology* 2007; 7(8):2930-2932.
[138] Bäumler H, Georgieva R. Coupled enzyme reactions in multicompartment microparticles. *Biomacromolecules* 2010; 11(6):1480-1487.
[139] Ballantyne B, Jordan SL. Toxicological, medical and industrial hygiene aspects of glutaraldehyde with particular reference to its biocidal use in cold sterilization procedures. *Journal of Applied Toxicology* 2001; 21(2):131-151.
[140] Zissu D, Bonnet P, Binet S. Histopathological study in B6C3F1 mice chronically exposed by inhalation to glutaraldehyde. *Toxicology Letters* 1998; 95(2):131-139.
[141] Iemma F, Spizzirri UG, Muzzalupo R, Puoci F, Trombino S, Picci N. Spherical hydrophilic microparticles obtained by the radical copolymerisation of functionalised bovine serum albumin. *Colloid and Polymer Science* 2004; 283(3):250-256.
[142] Iemma F, Spizzirri UG, Puoci F, Cirillo G, Curcio M, Parisi OI, Picci N. Synthesis and release profile analysis of thermo-sensitive albumin hydrogels. *Colloid and Polymer Science* 2009; 287(7):779-787.
[143] Iemma F, Spizzirri UG, Puoci F, Muzzalupo R, Trombino S, Cassano R, Leta S, Picci N. pH-Sensitive hydrogels based on bovine serum albumin for oral drug delivery. *International Journal of Pharmaceutics* 2006; 312(1-2):151-157.
[144] Cirillo G, Iemma F, Spizzirri UG, Puoci F, Curcio M, Parisi OI, Picci N. Synthesis of stimuli-responsive microgels for in vitro release of diclofenac diethyl ammonium. *Journal of Biomaterials Science, Polymer Edition* 2011; 22(4-6):823-844.
[145] Morgan PW, Kwolek SL. Interfacial polycondensation II; Fundamentals of polymer formation at liquid interfaces. *Journal of Polymer Science* 1959; 40:299.
[146] Chang TMS. Semipermeable microcapsules. *Science* 1964; 146(3643):524-525.
[147] Levy M-C, Lefebvre S, Rahmouni M, Andry M-C, Manfait M. Fourier transform infrared spectroscopic studies of human serum albumin microcapsules prepared by interfacial cross-linking with terephthaloylchloride: Influence of polycondensation pH on spectra and relation with microcapsule morphology and size. *Journal of Pharmaceutical Sciences* 1991; 80(6):578-585.

[148] Levy M-C, Lefebvre S, Andry M-C, Rahmouni M, Manfait M. Fourier-transform infrared spectroscopic studies of cross-linked human serum albumin microcapsules. 2. Influence of reaction time on spectra and correlation with microcapsule morphology and size. *Journal of Pharmaceutical Sciences* 1994; 83(3):419-422.

[149] Levy M-C, Lefebvre S, Andry M-C, Manfait M. Fourier transform infrared spectroscopic studies of cross-linked human serum albumin microcapsules. 3. Influence of terephthaloyl chloride concentration on spectra and correlation with microcapsule morphology and size. *Journal of Pharmaceutical Sciences* 1995; 84(2):161-165.

[150] Edwards-Levy F, Andry M-C, Levy M-C. Determination of free amino group content of serum albumin microcapsules using trinitrobenzenesulfonic acid: Effect of variations in polycondensation pH. *International Journal of Pharmaceutics* 1993; 96(1-3):85-90.

[151] Edwards-Lévy F, Andry M-C, Lévy M-C. Determination of free amino group content of serum albumin microcapsules: II. Effect of variations in reaction time and in terephthaloyl chloride concentration. *International Journal of Pharmaceutics* 1994; 103(3):253-257.

[152] Andry M-C, Edwards-Lévy F, Lévy M-C. Free amino group content of serum albumin microcapsules. III. A study at low pH values. *International Journal of Pharmaceutics* 1996; 128(1-2):197-202.

[153] Andry M-C, Lévy M-C. In vitro degradation of serum albumin microcapsules: Effect of process variables. *International Journal of Pharmaceutics* 1997; 152(2):145-151.

[154] Levy M-C, Andry M-C. Microcapsules prepared through interfacial cross-linking of starch derivatives. *International Journal of Pharmaceutics* 1990; 62(1):27-35.

[155] Hettler D, Andry M-C, Levy M-C. Polyhydroxamic microcapsules prepared from proteins: A novel type of chelating microcapsules. *Journal of Microencapsulation* 1994; 11(2):213-224.

[156] Levy M-C, Hettler D, Andry M-C, Rambourg P. Polyhydroxamic serum albumin microcapsules: Preparation and chelating properties. *International Journal of Pharmaceutics* 1991; 69(1):R1-R4.

[157] Pariot N, Edwards-Lévy F, Andry M-C, Lévy M-C. Cross-linked β-cyclodextrin microcapsules: Preparation and properties. *International Journal of Pharmaceutics* 2000; 211(1-2):19-27.

[158] Pariot N, Edwards-Lévy F, Andry M-C, Lévy M-C. Cross-linked β-cyclodextrin microcapsules. II. Retarding effect on drug release through semi-permeable membranes. *International Journal of Pharmaceutics* 2002; 232(1-2):175-181.

[159] Sawaya A, Benoit J-P, Benita S. Binding mechanism of doxorubicin in ion-exchange albumin microcapsules. *Journal of Pharmaceutical Sciences* 1987; 76(6):475-480.

[160] Larionova NV, Ponchel G, Duchêne D, Larionova NI. Biodegradable cross-linked starch/protein microcapsules containing proteinase inhibitor for oral protein administration. *International Journal of Pharmaceutics* 1999; 189(2):171-178.

[161] Krasota A, Belousova R, Duchêne D, Larionova N. In vitro inhibition of bovine herpes virus 1 reproduction with native and microencapsulated proteinase inhibitor aprotinin. *Journal of Controlled Release* 2002; 85(1-3):117-124.

[162] Edwards-Lévy F, Wurtz H. unpublished data.

[163] Levy M-C, Edwards-Levy F. Coating alginate beads with cross-linked biopolymers: A novel method based on a transacylation reaction. *Journal of Microencapsulation* 1996; 13(2):169-183.

[164] Vandamme TF, Poncelet D, Subra-Paternault P. Microencapsulation: des sciences aux technologies. Ed. Tec and Doc; Lavoisier 2007.
[165] Edwards-Lévy F, Lévy M-C. Serum albumin-alginate coated beads: Mechanical properties and stability. *Biomaterials* 1999; 20(21):2069-2084.
[166] Carin M, Barthès-Biesel D, Edwards-Lévy F, Postel C, Andrei DC. Compression of biocompatible liquid-filled HSA-alginate capsules: Determination of the membrane mechanical properties. *Biotechnology and Bioengineering* 2003; 82(2):207-212.
[167] Rachik M, Barthes-Biesel D, Carin M, F. Edwards-Levy. Identification of the elastic properties of an artificial capsule membrane with the compression test: Effect of thickness. *Journal of Colloid and Interface Science* 2006; 301(1):217-226.
[168] Sherwood JD, Risso F, Collé-Paillot F, Edwards-Lévy F, Lévy M-C. Rates of transport through a capsule membrane to attain Donnan equilibrium. *Journal of Colloid and Interface Science* 2003; 263(1):202-212.
[169] Lim F, Sun AM. Microencapsulated islets as bioartifical endocrine pancreas. *Science* 1980; 210(4472):908-910.
[170] Joly A, Desjardins J-F, Fremond B, Desille M, Campion J-P, Malledant Y, Lebreton Y, Semana G, Edwards-Levy F, Levy M-C, Clement B. Survival, proliferation, and functions of porcine hepatocytes encapsulated in coated alginate beads: A step toward a reliable bioartificial liver. *Transplantation* 1997; 63(6):795-803.
[171] Callewaert M, Laurent-Maquin D, Edwards-Lévy F. Albumin-alginate-coated microspheres: Resistance to steam sterilization and to lyophilization. *International Journal of Pharmaceutics* 2007; 344(1-2):161-164.
[172] Edwards-Lévy F, Munin A. unpublished data.
[173] Zaky A, Elbakry A, Ehmer A, Breunig M, Goepferich A. The mechanism of protein release from triglyceride microspheres. *Journal of Controlled Release* 2010; 147(2):202-210.
[174] Hua Z, Zhou S, Zhao M. Fabrication of a surface imprinted hydrogel shell over silica microspheres using bovine serum albumin as a model protein template. *Biosensors and Bioelectronics* 2009; 25(3):615-622.
[175] Saralidze K, Knetsch MLW, Van Der Marel C, Koole LH. Versatile polymer microspheres for injection therapy: Aspects of fluoroscopic traceability and biofunctionalization. *Biomacromolecules* 2010; 11(12):3556-3562.
[176] Brook MA, Jiang J, Heritage P, Bartzoka V, Underdown B, McDermott MR. Silicone-protein interaction at the interface between a functional silicone and a protein/starch microparticle. *Langmuir* 1997; 13(23):6279-6286.
[177] Brook MA, Jiang J, Heritage P, Underdown B, McDermott MR. Silicone-modified starch/protein microparticles: Protecting biopolymers with a hydrophobic coating. *Colloids and Surfaces B: Biointerfaces* 1997; 9(6):285-295.
[178] Péan JM, Venier-Julienne MC, Filmon R, Sergent M, Phan-Tan-Luu R, Benoit JP. Optimization of HSA and NGF encapsulation yields in PLGA microparticles. *International Journal of Pharmaceutics* 1998; 166(1):105-115.
[179] Bjerknes K, Dyrstad K, Smistad G, Agerkvist I. Preparation of polymeric microcapsules: Formulation studies. *Drug Development and Industrial Pharmacy* 2000; 26(8):847-856.

[180] Malzert-Fréon A, Schönhammer K, Benoît J-P, Boury F. Interactions between poly(ethylene glycol) and protein in dichloromethane/water emulsions. 2. Conditions required to obtain spontaneous emulsification allowing the formation of bioresorbable poly(d,l lactic acid) microparticles. *European Journal of Pharmaceutics and Biopharmaceutics* 2009; 73(1):66-73.

[181] Yeh M-K, Chen J-L, Chiang C-H, Chang Z-Y. The preparation of sustained release erythropoietin microparticle. *Journal of Microencapsulation* 2007; 24(1):82-93.

[182] Srinivasan C, Katare YK, Muthukumaran T, Panda AK. Effect of additives on encapsulation efficiency, stability and bioactivity of entrapped lysozyme from biodegradable polymer particles. *Journal of Microencapsulation* 2005; 22(2):127-138.

[183] Rafi M, Singh SM, Kanchan V, Anish CK, Panda AK. Controlled release of bioactive recombinant human growth hormone from PLGA microparticles. *Journal of Microencapsulation* 2010; 27(6):552-560.

[184] Schneider S, Feilen P, Cramer H, Hillgärtner M, Brunnenmeier F, Zimmermann H, Weber MM, Zimmermann U. Beneficial effects of human serum albumin on stability and functionality of alginate microcapsules fabricated in different ways. *Journal of Microencapsulation* 2003; 20(5):627-636.

[185] Lee J, Oh YJ, Lee SK, Lee KY. Facile control of porous structures of polymer microspheres using an osmotic agent for pulmonary delivery. *Journal of Controlled Release* 2010; 146(1):61-67.

[186] Rathod S, Deshpande S. Albumin microspheres as an ocular delivery system for pilocarpine nitrate. *Indian Journal of Pharmaceutical Sciences* 2008; 70(2):193-197.

[187] Ying X, Zhang F, Zhang L, Cheng G. Effect on rebinding behavior with different composition and structure of the dually imprinted alginate polymer microspheres using proteins and o/w emulsion drops as dual templates. *J. Appl. Polym. Sci.* 2010; 115(6):3516-3526.

[188] Lefebvre Y, Leclerc E, Barthès-Biesel D, Walter J, Edwards-Lévy F. Flow of artificial microcapsules in microfluidic channels: A method for determining the elastic properties of the membrane. *Physics of Fluids* 2008; 20(12):123102.

[189] Chu TX, Salsac A-V, Leclerc E, Barthès-Biesel D, Wurtz H, Edwards-Lévy F. Comparison between measurements of elasticity and free amino group content of ovalbumin microcapsule membranes: Discrimination of the cross-linking degree. *Journal of Colloid and Interface Science* 2011; 355(1):81-88.

[190] Coombes AGA, Breeze V, Lin W, Gray T, Parker KG, Parker T. Lactic acid-stabilised albumin for microsphere formulation and biomedical coatings. *Biomaterials* 2001; 22(1):1-8.

In: Serum Albumin: Structure, Functions and Health Impact ISBN: 978-1-62100-231-4
Editors: R. J. Alekseev and A. L. Rebane

Chapter 4

ANALYSIS OF HYDRATION OF HUMAN SERUM ALBUMIN BY ISOTHERMAL CALORIMETRY

Vladimir A. Sirotkin*
Kazan (Volga Region) Federal University, A.M. Butlerov Chemical Institute, Kazan, Russia

ABSTRACT

This work describes the basic principles of a novel experimental approach for studying the hydration of proteins. This method, based on the calorimetric measurements, allows for the simultaneous monitoring of the excess partial enthalpies of water and the protein obtained in the entire range of water contents. Human serum albumin (HSA) was used as a model protein.

The excess partial quantities of water and HSA are very sensitive to the hydration level. At the lowest water contents, HSA is in a rigid (glassy) state. Changes of the excess thermochemical function can mainly be attributed to water addition.

A transition from the glassy to the flexible state of HSA is accompanied by significant changes in the excess partial quantities of water and HSA. This transition appears at water weight fraction (w_1) of 0.06 when charged and polar groups of HSA are covered.

Excess partial quantities reach their fully hydrated values at $w_1 > 0.4$ when coverage of both polar and weakly interacting surface elements is complete. At the highest water contents, water addition has no significant effect on the excess thermochemical function. At $w_1 > 0.4$, the observed changes in the excess function can solely be attributed to changes in the protein structure.

1. BACKGROUND AND SIGNIFICANCE

The hydration of proteins is a phenomenon of considerable fundamental importance and practical interest. It is well known that water bound to proteins (hydration or biological water)

* E-mail: vsir@mail.ru, Personal site: http://vsirotkin2006.narod.ru/Sirotkin_engl_2009.html

2. Methodology

The correct analysis of the thermochemical data requires the definition of the system under study. The first consideration is the case when:

(1) Initially, the solid protein phase does not contain water.

(2) The transfer of water from the gas phase to the protein phase occurs at 25 °C and atmospheric pressure. Then, the enthalpy change corresponding to the mixing of the dried protein with water is given by Eq. 3:

$$\Delta H_{\text{Solid-Gas}}(\text{dried}) = [\overline{H}_W m_W]_{\text{final solid}} + [\overline{H}_W m_W]_{\text{final gas}} + [\overline{H}^h_P m_P]_{\text{final solid}} - [\overline{H}_W m_W]_{\text{initial gas}} - [\overline{H}^0_P m_P]_{\text{initial solid}} \quad (3)$$

$\overline{H}_P$ and $\overline{H}_W$ are the partial enthalpies of the protein and water, respectively; and where m_P, m_W are mass amounts of the protein and water, respectively. Phases (gas or solid) and states (final or initial) are specified by subscripts. The amount of water, m_W^{tr}, transferred from the gas phase to the protein phase is defined as in Eq. 4:

$$m_W^{tr} = [m_{W,\text{final}} - m_{W,\text{initial}}]_{\text{solid}} = [m_{W,\text{initial}} - m_{W,\text{final}}]_{\text{gas}} = m_{W,\text{final..solid}} \quad (4)$$

The partial enthalpy of water in the gas phase is not changed during the interaction with the protein. Therefore, Eq. 3 can be transformed into Eq. 5:

$$\begin{aligned} &\Delta H_{\text{Solid-Gas}}(\text{dried}) = [\overline{H}_{P,\text{final}} - \overline{H}_{P,\text{initial}}]_{\text{solid}} * m_P \\ &[\overline{H}_W m_W]_{\text{solid}} + \overline{H}_{W,\text{gas}}[m_{W,\text{final gas}} - m_{W,\text{initial gas}}] = \\ &[\overline{H}^h_{P,\text{final}} - \overline{H}^0_{P,\text{initial}}]_{\text{solid}} * m_P + [\overline{H}_{W,\text{solid}} - \overline{H}_{W,\text{gas}}] m_W^{tr} \end{aligned} \quad (5)$$

The hydration of proteins can be characterized by two different methods.

Method 1. This is a typical way. The $\Delta H_{\text{Solid-Gas}}(\text{dried})$ value is related to the amount of water bound to the protein, m_W^h, (Eq. 6):

$$\Delta H_{\text{hydr}}^{H_2O/\text{gas}} = [\overline{H^h_P} - \overline{H^0_P}]_{\text{solid}} \frac{m_E}{m_W^h} + [\overline{H}_{W,\text{solid}} - \overline{H}_{W,\text{gas}}] \quad (6)$$

The $\Delta H_{\text{hydr}}^{H_2O/\text{gas}}$ value is called sometimes the enthalpy of protein hydration. As can be concluded from Eq. 6, *Method 1* does not allow for studying separately the protein and water enthalpic contributions to the calorimetrically measured heat effects. According to Eq. 6, the $\Delta H_{hydr}^{H_2O/gas}$ value contains two components. The first component, $[\overline{H_P^h} - \overline{H_P^0}]_{solid} \frac{m_P}{m_w^h}$, is due to changes in the protein state during hydration (including conformational rearrangements and glass transition). The second component, $[\overline{H}_{w,solid} - \overline{H}_{w,gas}]$, is due to the difference between the water state in the gas phase and the bound state.

Method 2. The $\Delta H_{Solid\text{-}Gas}$ (dried) value observed during the addition of water to protein can be considered as an excess quantity of the mixing of water with protein (Z^E, Eq 1 and 2). From this quantity the excess partial enthalpies can be calculated using Eq. 7 and 8:

$$\overline{Z}_1^E = Z^E - w_2\left(\frac{\partial Z^E}{\partial w_2}\right)_{T,P} = [\overline{H}_{w,solid} - \overline{H}_{w,gas}] = \overline{H}_1^E \quad (7)$$

$$\overline{Z}_2^E = Z^E - w_1\left(\frac{\partial Z^E}{\partial w_1}\right)_{T,P} = [\overline{H_P^h} - \overline{H_P^0}]_{solid} = \overline{H}_2^E \quad (8)$$

where $\overline{H}_1^E$ and $\overline{H}_2^E$ are the excess partial enthalpies of water and protein, respectively; w_1 and w_2 are the mass fractions of water and protein, respectively. As can be concluded from Eq. 7 and 8, *Method 2* allows for studying separately the protein and water contributions to the calorimetrically measured heat effects.

Eq. 5 can be transformed into an expression useful for experimental applications. When the transfer of water from the liquid phase to the protein phase occurs, Eq. 5 can be transformed into Eq. 9:

$$\Delta H_{Solid\text{-}Liquid}(\text{dried}) = [\overline{H_{P,final}^h} - \overline{H}_{P,initial}^o]_{solid} m_P + [\overline{H}_{w,solid} - \overline{H}_{w,liquid}] m_w^{tr} \quad (9)$$

The enthalpy change corresponding to introducing some amount of protein in pure liquid water (the solution enthalpy, $\Delta_{sol} H$) can be defined by Eq. 10 and 11. Let's consider two variants. In both cases, the final state of the protein is a diluted solution in water at 25°C and atmospheric pressure.

Variant 1. Initially, the solid protein does not contain water.

$$\Delta_{sol} H\,(\text{dried}) = [\overline{H_P^b} m_P]_{final\ liquid} + [\overline{H}_w^b m_w^b]_{final\ protein} - [\overline{H}_w m_w^b]_{initial\ liquid} - [\overline{H}_P^o m_P]_{initial\ protein} \quad (10)$$

where $\overline{H}_W^b$ is the partial enthalpy of water bound to the protein in the solution; $\overline{H}_P^b$ is the partial enthalpy of the protein in the solution. m_W^b - is the amount of water bound to the protein in the solution.

Variant 2. The initial protein phase may contain water.

$$\Delta_{sol} H\,(\text{hydrated}) = [\overline{H}_W m_W^h]_{\text{final liquid}} + [\overline{H}_P^b m_P]_{\text{final liquid}} + [\overline{H}_W^b m_W^b]_{\text{final protein}} - [\overline{H}_W m_W^b]_{\text{initial liquid}} - [\overline{H}_P^h m_P + \overline{H}_W m_W^h]_{\text{initial protein}} \quad (11)$$

where $\overline{H}_P$ and $\overline{H}_W$ are the partial enthalpies of the protein and water; m_W^h is the amount of water bound to initial solid protein. m_W^b is the amount of water bound to the protein in the solution.

The amount of water transferred from the liquid phase to the protein phase is defined by Eq. 12, when the initial protein does not contain water:

$$m_W^{tr} = m_W^b \quad (12)$$

The amount of water transferred from the liquid phase to the protein phase is defined by Eq. 13, when the initial protein contains water:

$$m_W^{tr} = [m^b_{W,\text{final..protein}} - m^h_{W,\text{initial..protein}}] \quad (13)$$

The difference between the solution enthalpies for the dried and hydrated protein is defined by Eq. 14. It is expected that the partial enthalpy of water in liquid phase does not change significantly during the formation of the diluted protein solution.

$$\frac{\Delta_{sol} H\,(\text{dried}) - \Delta_{sol} H\,(\text{hydrated})}{m_W^h} = [\overline{H_P^h} - \overline{H_P^0}]_{\text{solid}} \frac{m_P}{m_W^h} + [\overline{H}_{W,\text{solid}} - \overline{H}_{W,\text{liquid}}] = \frac{\Delta H_{\text{Solid-Gas}}(\text{dried})}{m_W^h} + [\overline{H}_{W,\text{gas}} - \overline{H}_{W,\text{liquid}}] = \frac{\Delta H_{\text{Solid-Gas}}(\text{dried})}{m_W^h} + \Delta H_{vap}^{H_2O} \quad (14)$$

where $\Delta H_{vap}^{H_2O}$ is the enthalpy of vaporization of water (43.7 kJ mol^{-1}) [19].

As can be concluded from Eq. 14, the Z^E value (Eq. 1, 2, 7, and 8) can be calculated from the enthalpies of solution of the dried, $\Delta_{sol} H\,(\text{dried})$, and hydrated, $\Delta_{sol} H\,(\text{hydrated})$, protein in water measured by isothermal calorimetry.

Eq. 15 is similar to Eq. 2. It allows for calculating the excess partial quantities from the calorimetrically measured heat effects.

$$\frac{\Delta_{sol} H(\text{dried}) - \Delta_{sol} H(\text{hydrated})}{m_w^h + m_P} =$$
$$= [\overline{H_P^h} - \overline{H_P^0}]_{solid} \frac{m_P}{m_P + m_w^h} + [\overline{H}_{w,.solid} - \overline{H}_{w,.liquid}] \frac{m_w^h}{m_P + m_w^h} = \quad (15)$$
$$= [\overline{H_P^h} - \overline{H_P^0}]_{solid} w_2 + [\overline{H}_{w,.solid} - \overline{H}_{w,.liquid}] w_1$$

3. EXPERIMENTAL

Calorimetric experiments were conducted following the procedures described in detail elsewhere [20,21]. The enthalpy changes on the immersion of the dried protein into pure liquid water were measured at 25 °C with a Setaram BT-2.15 calorimeter according to the described procedure [20,21]. Typically, the sample of 8-10 mg of protein preparation contacted with 4.0 ml of water in the calorimetric cell. A typical time of a calorimetric experiment was about 40 min. A typical heat evolution curve recorded upon dissolution of solid HSA in pure liquid water is given in [21]. Calorimeter was calibrated using the Joule effect and tested with dissolving sodium chloride in water according to the recommendations [20].

The dried protein preparation (*zero hydration level*) was obtained by drying under vacuum using a microthermoanalyzer "Setaram" MGDTD-17S at 25 °C and 0.1 Pa until the constant sample weight was reached. Water content of the dried protein was estimated as 0.003 ± 0.002 g g^{-1} by the Karl Fischer titration method according to the recommendations [20].

At the lowest water activity (a_w) values, protein samples for the determination of the interaction enthalpies with water were equilibrated at 25±0.5 °C in tightly closed desiccator over saturated salt solutions. Water activities over saturated salt solutions were taken from [19]. The following salts were used: LiBr (a_w=0.064), KOH (a_w=0.078), LiCl (a_w=0.11), $CaBr_2$ (a_w=0.17), CH_3COOK (a_w=0.22), $MgCl_2$ (a_w=0.33), K_2CO_3 (a_w=0.44), $Mg(NO_3)_2$ (a_w=0.53), NaCl (a_w=0.75), KCl (a_w=0.84), KNO_3 (a_w=0.94). Salts for the conditioning of the samples were of analytical pure grade. The conditioned samples were then taken from the desiccator and equilibrated in the calorimetric cell at 25 °C before the experiment. Transfer of protein samples from dessicator into calorimetric cell was performed in the closed box with the varied water activity.

At the highest a_w values, the protein and water samples were mixed in the calorimetric cell at various water weight fractions and 25 °C. The masses of protein samples used in the equilibration were in the range 8-10 mg. Water content of the samples after equilibration was measured by drying under vacuum using a microthermoanalyzer "Setaram" MGDTD-17S at 25 °C and 0.1 Pa until the constant sample weight was reached.

4. Excess Partial Quantitites

4.1. Excess Partial Enthalpies of Water and Albumin

Figure 1 shows how the $\frac{\Delta_{sol} H(\text{hydrated}) - \Delta_{sol} H(\text{dried})}{m_w^h + m_P}$ values (excess function of mixing per unit mass of the mixture) depend on the hydration level of HSA. The initial state (zero hydration level) for studying the enthalpy of solution of the dried HSA in pure liquid water, $\Delta_{sol} H(\text{dried})$, was obtained by drying in air at a water activity less than 0.01. On maintaining this "dry" sample in equilibrium with a vacuum of 0.1 Pa and at 25 °C for three hours, it lost about 0.3 % of its weight, which for HSA implies that at the zero hydration level there are about 11 water molecules strongly bound to each protein molecule. The $\Delta_{sol} H(\text{dried})$ value is -8322 (125) kJ mol^{-1} or -126.1 (1.9) J g^{-1} HSA at 25°C.

Figure 2 and 3 present the excess partial enthalpy of water, $\overline{H}_1^E$, and the excess partial enthalpy of HSA, $\overline{H}_2^E$, as functions of the weight fraction of water. These thermochemical quantities were calculated using Eq. 7, 8, and 15. The enthalpy curves presented in Figure 4 and 5 can be divided into three parts.

Part 1. w_1=0-0.06 (h~0-0.07 g g^{-1}). The main features of part 1 can be described as follows. At the lowest water contents, the protein is in a glassy (rigid) state [1,13]. In the low water content range (w_1<0.06), the strong hydration sites are preferentially occupied [2]. Hutchens et al. [23] studied the heat capacities of chymotrypsinogen A at w_1 of 0 and 0.096, from -263 to 37 °C. No phase transition corresponding to the ice-liquid water transition was observed at low hydrations.

The excess partial enthalpy of water, $\overline{H}_1^E$, is highly exothermic (negative). The $\overline{H}_1^E$ value does not depend noticeably on the water content and equals approx. -61.5 kJ mol^{-1} water (Figure 2). The excess partial enthalpy of HSA, $\overline{H}_2^E$, is close to zero (Figure 3). The $\overline{H}_2^E$ value does not depend noticeably on the water content. The fact that HSA is in the glassy state explains this feature of part 1. The $\overline{H}_2^E$ value is rather constant due to the fact that all the protein molecules came into contact mainly with the same protein molecules during this range of water contents.

Certain conclusions regarding the nature of the water sorption sites of the dehydrated protein can be made by analyzing the excess partial enthalpies of water in various organic solvents. The $\overline{H}_1^E$ (w_1=0) value for HSA was compared with the enthalpies of solvation of water in organic solvents at infinite dilution, $\Delta_{solv} H^{H_2O/S}$, in Table 1. The enthalpy of solvation, $\Delta_{solv} H^{A/S}$, is the enthalpy of isothermal transfer of solute A (H_2O) from the ideal gas state to an infinitively diluted solution in solvent S (organic solvent) at 25 °C and 0.1 MPa. The solution enthalpy, $\Delta_{sol} H^{A/S}$, is the enthalpy of transfer of solute A from its standard state (solid, liquid or gas) to an infinitively diluted solution in solvent S at 25 °C and 0.1 MPa. Solvation and solution enthalpies are interrelated through Eq. 16:

$$\Delta_{solv} H^{H_2O/S} = \Delta_{sol} H^{H_2O/S} - \Delta H_{vap}^{H_2O} =$$
$$= [\overline{H}_{w,org\,S} - \overline{H}_{w,liquid}] - [\overline{H}_{w,gas} - \overline{H}_{w,liquid}] = \qquad (16)$$
$$= \overline{H}_{w,org\,S} - \overline{H}_{w,gas}$$

where $\Delta_{sol} H^{H_2O/S}$ is the enthalpy of solution of water in organic solvent, kJ mol^{-1}; $\Delta H_{vap}^{H_2O}$ is the enthalpy of vaporization of water, 43.7 kJ mol^{-1}.

$$H^E - x_2\left(\frac{\partial H^E}{\partial x_2}\right)_{T,P} = \overline{H}_1^E \qquad (17)$$

where H^E is the excess enthalpy of mixing; $\overline{H}_1^E$ is the excess partial enthalpy of water in organic solvent; x_2 is the mol fraction of organic solvent.

The $\Delta_{sol} H^{H_2O/S}$ values were estimated using Eq. 18:

$$\Delta_{sol} H^{H_2O/S} = \overline{H}_1^E - \overline{H}_1^o \qquad (18)$$

where $\overline{H}_1^o$ is the partial enthalpy of water in the standard state (pure liquid water at 25 °C and 0.1 MPa). The H^E values for water-organic mixtures were taken from [24,25].

Diethylamine, acetic acid, ethanol and N,N-dimethylformamide (DMFA) were used as analogues of various protein groups. Acetic acid was used as an analogue of the amino acids containing the side carboxylic groups. Diethylamine was used as an analogue of the amino acids containing the side amino groups. DMFA was used a low molecular analogue of the polypeptide backbone. Ethanol was used as an analogue of the amino acids containing the side OH groups.

As can be concluded from Table 1, the $\overline{H}_1^E$ value is close to that observed for diethylamine which has the most exothermic excess partial enthalpy of water from the solvents under study (-58.1 kJ mol^{-1}). This result suggests that, at the lowest w_1 values, the interaction with the amino groups may be a dominant factor controlling the state of water molecules.

Table 1. Enthalpies of solvation of water in organic solvents at infinite dilution and 25 °C.[a]

Solvent	$\Delta_{solv} H^{H_2O/S}$, kJ mol^{-1}
Diethylamine	-58.1 (18°C) [24]
Acetic acid	-40.9 [25]
N,N- dimethylformamide	-47.4 [25]
Ethanol	-45.7 [25]

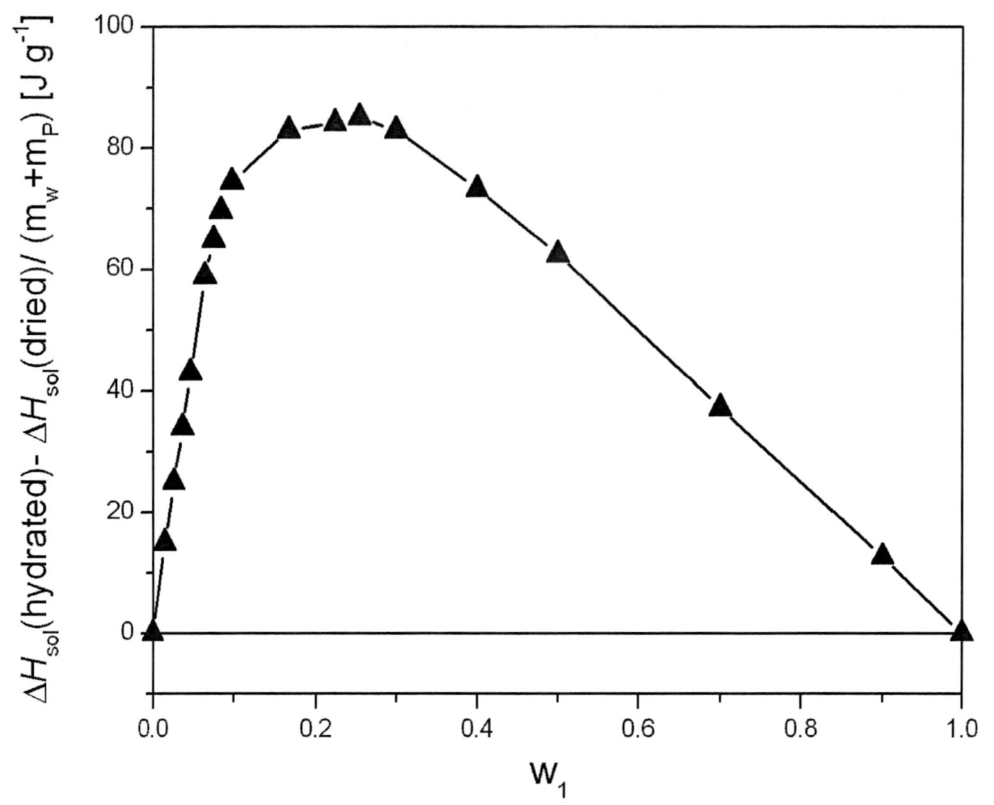

Figure 1. The $\frac{\Delta_{sol} H\text{(hydrated)} - \Delta_{sol} H\text{(dried)}}{m_w^h + m_P}$ value as a function of the weight fraction of water, w1, at 25 oC. Standard errors of estimation of the $\frac{\Delta_{sol} H\text{(hydrated)} - \Delta_{sol} H\text{(dried)}}{m_w^h + m_P}$ values were 1-2 J g-1 mixture.

Part 2. w_1=0.06-0.4. The main features of part 2 are the following. During isothermal sorption of water, a glasslike transition results in a step on the excess partial enthalpy of water (protein) curve (Figure 2 and 3). $\overline{H}_1^E$ decreases from highly negative to moderate values. $\overline{H}_2^E$ increases from very low values to highly exothermic values. There are two steps on the $\overline{H}_1^E$-w_1 and $\overline{H}_2^E$-w_1 curves. In the water content interval of w_1 ~ 0.06-0.2, the $\overline{H}_1^E$ and $\overline{H}_2^E$ values change sharply. In water content interval of w_1 ~ 0.2-0.4, the $\overline{H}_1^E$ and $\overline{H}_2^E$ values change moderately.

Apparent heat capacity of lysozyme, ϕC_{p2}, determined from isothermal experiments using a drop calorimeter increases from very low values to high values in this water content interval

[7]. This strong increase of the heat capacity was interpreted in terms of a transition of the protein molecules from a glassy (rigid) state to a flexible (elastic) state [13].

The results obtained for proteins and biopolymers by several experimental methods have been summarised in Ref. [1]. It was concluded that proteins undergo a glasslike transition at water content of about 10 wt% at 25 °C. This water content is within part 2 in this work.

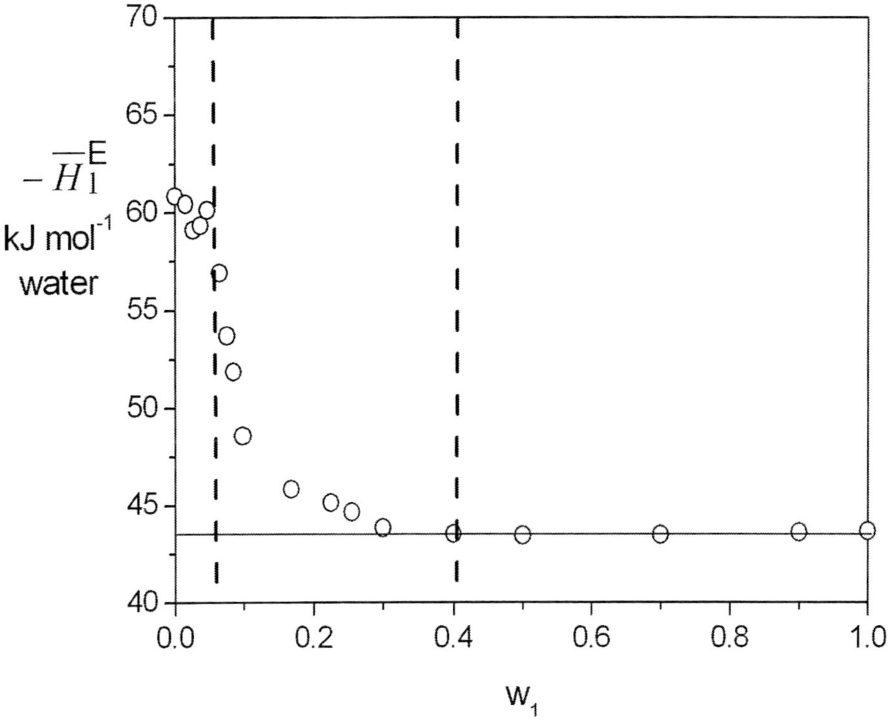

Figure 2. Excess partial enthalpy of water, $\overline{H}_1^E$, as a function of the weight fraction of water, w_1, at 25°C. Excess partial enthalpy of water was corrected for the enthalpy of condensation of water at 25 °C.

Part 3. $w_1 > 0.4$. The main features of part 3 can be described as follows. At the highest water contents (w_1>0.4), the protein is in a flexible (elastic) state [1, 13]. The structural rearrangements are largely completed [1]. Excess partial quantities reach their fully hydrated values at water weight fraction more than 0.4 when coverage of both polar and adjacent weakly interacting surface elements no longer changes appreciably upon further hydration. The $\overline{H}_1^E$ value is close to the enthalpy of condensation of pure water at 25 °C and atmospheric pressure (-43.7 kJ mol^{-1}). This implies that the average state of water in the hydrated HSA is close to that in the pure liquid water. Apparent heat capacity of lysozyme, ϕC_{p2}, [7] and excess partial enthalpy of HSA, $\overline{H}_2^E$, (Figure 3) reach their maximal values. This means that all the protein molecules are in the flexible state.

CONCLUSIONS

Isothermal butch calorimetry was applied to study the hydration of human serum albumin. The hydration process was characterized by a novel method based on the analysis of the excess partial quantities. This method allows for studying separately the protein and water excess partial quantities in the entire range of water content.

It was shown that the excess partial quantities of water and human serum albumin are very sensitive to the hydration level. At the lowest water contents, HSA is in a rigid (glassy) state. Changes of the excess thermochemical function can mainly be attributed to water addition.

A transition from the glassy to the flexible state of HSA is accompanied by significant changes in the excess partial quantities of water and human serum albumin. This transition appears in the calculated quantities when charged groups of HSA are covered, which occurs at a water weight fraction of 0.06 and 25 ^{o}C.

Excess partial quantities reach their fully hydrated values at a water weight fraction more than 0.4 when coverage of both polar and adjacent weakly interacting surface elements no longer changes appreciably upon further hydration. At $w_1 > 0.4$, the observed changes in the excess function can solely be attributed to changes in the protein structure.

REFERENCES

[1] Gregory, R.B. Protein hydration and glass transition behavior. In: Gregory, R.B., editor. *Protein-Solvent Interactions*, Marcel Dekker, New York, 1995, 191-264.

[2] Rupley, J.A., Careri, G. Protein hydration and function, *Adv. Protein Chem.* 1991, 41, 37-172.

[3] Mattos, C. Protein-water interactions in a dynamic world, *Trends. Biochem. Sci.* 2002, 27, 203-208.

[4] Kuntz, I.D., Kauzmann, W. Hydration of proteins and polypeptides., *Adv. Protein. Chem.* 1974, 28, 239-345.

[5] Nakasako, M. Water-protein interactions from high-resolution protein crystallography, *Philos. Trans. R. Soc. B.* 2004, 359, 1191-1204.

[6] Yang, P.-H., Rupley, J.A Protein-water interactions. Heat capacity of the lysozyme-water system. *Biochemistry* 1979, 18, 2654-2661.

[7] Luscher-Mattli, M., Ruegg, M. Thermodynamic functions of biopolymer hydration. I. Their determination by vapor pressure studies, discussed in an analysis of the primary hydration process. *Biopolymers* 1982, 21, 403-418.

[8] Luscher-Mattli, M., Ruegg, M. Thermodynamic functions of biopolymer hydration. II. Enthalpy-entropy compensation i8n hydrophilic hydration process. *Biopolymers* 1982, 21, 419-429.

[9] Bone, S. Dielectric and gravimetric studies of water binding to lysozyme. *Phys. Med. Biol.* 1996, 41, 1265-1275.

[10] Hnojewyj, W.S., Reyerson, L.H. Further studies on the sorption of H_2O and D_2O vapors by lysozyme and the deuterium-hydrogen exchange effect. *J. Phys. Chem.* 1961, 65, 1694-1698.

[11] Amberg, Heats of adsorption of water vapor on bovine serum albumin. *J. Amer. Chem. Soc.* 1957, 79, 3980-3984.

[12] Smith, A.L., Shirazi, H. M., Mulligan, S. R. Water sorption isotherms and enthalpies of water sorption by lysozyme using the quartz crystal microbalance/heat conduction calorimeter. *Biochim. Biophys. Acta,* 2002, 1594, 150-159.

[13] Kocherbitov, V., Arnebrant, T., Söderman, O. Lysozyme-water interactions studied by sorption calorimetry. *J. Phys. Chem. B.* 2004, 108, 19036-19042.

[14] Sirotkin, V.A., Korolev, D.V., Silakova, A.E. Hydration-dehydration of human serum albumin studied by isothermal calorimetry and IR spectroscopy. *Russ. J. Phys. Chem. A.* 2007, 81, 1341-1345.

[15] Sirotkin, V.A., Korolev, D.V. Effect of acetonitrile on the hydration of human serum albumin films. *Thermochim. Acta*, 2005, 432, 246-253.

[16] Sirotkin, V.A., Faizullin, D.A. Interaction enthalpies of solid human serum albumin with water-dioxane mixtures: comparison with water and organic solvent vapor sorption. *Thermochim. Acta*, 2004, 415, 127-133.

[17] Yu, X., Park, J., Leitner, D. M. Thermodynamics of protein hydration computed by molecular dynamics and normal modes. *J. Phys. Chem. B,* 2003, 107, 12820-12829.

[18] Carter, D.C., Ho, J.X. Structure of serum albumin, *Adv. Prot. Chem.* 1994, 45, 153-203.

[19] Nikol'skii, B.P. *Spravochnik Khimika (Chemist's Handbook)*, Leningrad, Goskhimizdat, 1963.

[20] Borisover, M.D., Sirotkin, V.A., Zakharychev, D.V., Solomonov, B.N. Calorimetric methods in evaluating hydration and solvation of solid proteins immersed in organic solvents, In: Vulfson, E.N., Halling, P.J., editors. *Enzymes in Nonaqueous Solvents*, Humana Press, Totowa, 2001, 183-202.

[21] Sirotkin, V.A., Zinatullin, A.N., Solomonov, B.N., Faizullin, D.A., Fedotov, V.D. Calorimetric and Fourier transform infrared spectroscopic study of solid proteins immersed in low water organic solvents, *Biochim. Biophys. Acta*, 2001, 1547, 359-369.

[22] Sirotkin, V.A., Analysis of the organic solvent effect on the hydration-dehydration and structure of proteins by FTIR spectroscopy, In: Uversky, V.N., Permyakov, E.N., editors. *Methods in Protein Structure and Stability Analysis: Vibrational spectroscopy,* Nova Science Publishers, Inc., Hauppauge, NY. 2007, 195-230.

[23] Hutchens, J. O., Cole, A.G. Stout, J.W. Heat capacities from 11 to 305 K and entropies of hydrated and anhydrous bovine zinc insulin and bovine chymotrypsinogen A. *J. Biol. Chem.* 1969, 244, 26-32.

[24] Bittrich H.-J., Kraft G., Mischungsenthalpien im System Diäthylamin – Wasser. *Z. Phys. Chem.* (Leipzig), 1964, 227, 359-370.

[25] Belousov, V.P., Morachevski, A.G., *Heats of Mixing of Liquids*, Khimiya, Leningrad, 1970.

In: Serum Albumin: Structure, Functions and Health Impact ISBN: 978-1-62100-231-4
Editors: R. J. Alekseev and A. L. Rebane

Chapter 5

INVESTIGATION OF DENATURATION OF HUMAN SERUM ALBUMIN UNDER ACTION OF IONIC SURFACTANTS BY ANALYSIS OF TRYPTOPHAN FLUORESCENCE OF PROTEIN

Irina M. Vlasova *

Russia, Moscow, 119991, M.V. Lomonosov Moscow State University, Department of Physics

ABSTRACT

The tryptophan fluorescence of human serum albumin (HSA) at addition of ionic surfactants (anionic surfactant sodium dodecyl sulfate SDS and cationic surfactant cethyltrimethylammonium bromide CTAB) in protein solution at various values of pH was investigated, what gave information about mechanism of denaturation of HSA under action of ionic surfactants. The analysis of non-polarized and polarized steady-state tryptophan fluorescence of HSA in solutions with SDS and CTAB was done.

The experimental dependences of intensity and polarization of tryptophan fluorescence of HSA on concentrations of SDS (0 – 7 mM) and CTAB (0 – 7 mM) in solutions at various values of pH (3.5 – 8.0) were found out. The quenching of tryptophan fluorescence of HSA in solutions with ionic surfactants was registered, and the value of this quenching depends not only on concentration of surfactant, but also on value of pH. The polarization of tryptophan fluorescence of HSA in solutions with ionic surfactants increases.

The calculation of parameters of rotational diffusion (coefficient of rotational diffusion, time of rotational relaxation and effective Einstein's radius) of HSA molecules in solutions with various concentrations of SDS and CTAB at various values of pH was done. In solutions with ionic surfactants SDS and CTAB the decrease of coefficient of rotational diffusion of HSA, the increase of time of rotational relaxation of HSA, corresponding to disordering owing to thermal diffusion, and the increase of effective Einstein's radius of HSA molecules take place, what speaks about denaturation of HSA

*Tel.: +74959391489 Fax: +74959391489, E-mail: vlasovairina1979@mail.ru

under action of these ionic surfactants – decondensation of protein globules with increase of its linear-longitude sizes and unfolding of amino-acidic chain of protein.

On basis of received dependences the conclusion was done, that denaturation of HSA under action of cationic surfactant CTAB has one-stage character at all investigated values of pH, but denaturation of HSA under action of anionic surfactant SDS has more complex character – at values of pH, lower than pI of HSA, denaturation has two stage-character, and at values of pH, higher than pI of HSA, denaturation has one-stage character. It is shown that more deep denaturation of HSA under action of CTAB takes place at values of pH, higher than pI of HSA, on contrary more deep denaturation of HSA under action of SDS takes place at values of pH, lower than pI of HSA.

Keywords: human serum albumin, tryptophan, fluorescence, ionic surfactant, sodium dodecyl sulfate, cethyltrimethylammonium bromide

1. Introduction

The human serum albumin (molecular mass 66.4 kDa, isoelectric point pI 4.7) is the globular protein of human blood plasma. Unique property of molecule of human serum albumin (HSA) to bind many types of organic and inorganic ligands determines one of fundamental functions of this protein – the transport of physiological metabolites and drugs.

The structural mobility of HSA molecule, provided by unique loop folding of one polypeptide chain of 585 amino-acidic residues, ensures the interaction of HSA molecule with ligands [1]. The secondary structure of HSA, stabilized by hydrogen bonds between peptide groups of amino-acidic chain, consists of α-helical segments and segments of random packing (random clew). About 50 – 67 % of amino-acidic residues of HSA are folded in the α-helices at physiological value of pH. In non-helical segments the protein chain is bent. Between amino-acidic residues of Cysteine in HSA the 17 disulfide bonds are formed which form 9 loops, or subdomains (6 large and 3 small loops). The structural unit, containing 2 large loops and 1 small loop, represents globular structure named the domain. Nowadays the domain model of HSA structure is accepted, according to which the molecule of HSA consists of 3 practically identical domains, the domains in this model are arranged at some angle to each other (tertiary structure of HSA is in the form of "heart"). Stability of tertiary structure depends not only on system non-covalent interactions in protein globule, but also on covalent disulfide bonds. Denaturation is the essential change of secondary and tertiary structure of protein, i.e. the disturbance and un-regulation of system of non-covalent interactions, without influence on protein covalent structure. The denaturation, as a rule, is accompanied by loss of functional properties of protein what causes the interest to analysis of mechanisms of protein denaturation. The effective agents, induced denaturation, are the ionic surfactants. The surfactants (detergents) represent organic amphiphilic compounds which molecules have hydrophilic and hydrophobic segments. On type of hydrophilic groups one can divide surfactants into ionic and non-ionic. Ionic surfactants in solution dissociate on the ions one of which are surface-active, and others (anti-ions) - are not surface-active. Depending on a sign of charge of surface-active ion the ionic surfactants are separated on anionic, cationic and amphoteric [2, 3]. Ionic surfactants, having denaturating properties, are very popular in pharmaceutical, medical and biochemical researches. Among them are the anionic surfactant sodium dodecyl sulfate (SDS), often used in electrophoretic researches, and the cationic surfactant cethyltrimethylammonium bromide (CTAB) with bactericidal properties and activity against Gram-positive and Gram-negative bacteria (at alkaline values of pH) [2, 3]. Investigation of tryptophan intrinsic fluorescence of proteins is widely applied for an estimation of conformational state of protein molecules [4-9]. Unique amino-acidic residue of tryptophan (Trp-214) in HSA is located in the domain II. Fluorescence properties of tryptophan in HSA molecule are rather sensitive to rearrangements of protein globule.

The investigation of denaturation of HSA under action of anionic surfactant SDS and cationic surfactant CTAB is important due to the physiological functions of HSA in blood, it allows one to make conclusions about level of safety of native conformation of protein and, hence, about safety of its physiological properties in various conditions.

Earlier in my articles the investigations of denaturation of HSA under action of SDS [10-14] and CTAB [15, 16] were done by various spectroscopic methods – laser correlation spectroscopy, Raman spectroscopy and fluorescent analysis with use of nanomarker eosin.

In this work the investigations of mechanism of denaturation of HSA under action of various concentrations of SDS and CTAB at various values of pH were done with the help of fluorescent analysis of intrinsic tryptophan fluorescence of HSA.

2. Materials and Methods

The following buffer solutions were prepared: 0.1 M CH_3COOH – KOH, pH (3.0 – 5.0) and 0.1 M KH_2PO_4 – 0.1 M NaOH, pH (6.0 – 8.0). HSA was diluted in buffer solutions up to concentration 5 μM. In the first case the different concentrations of SDS (0.5 – 7.0 mM) were added in HSA solutions at various values of pH (3.5 – 6.0). In the second case the different concentrations of CTAB (0.5 – 7.0 mM) were added in HSA solutions at various values of pH (3.5 – 8.0). For the analysis of rotational diffusion of HSA molecules in final protein solutions with surfactants the various concentrations of sucrose (0 – 200 mM) were added.

Fluorescent investigations of samples were made with the help of spectrofluorimeter LS 55 (Perkin Elmer) at room temperature. Spectra of tryptophan fluorescence of HSA were registered in the range 300 – 500 nm at excitation by light with wavelength λ_{exc} = 295 nm. The degree of polarization P of tryptophan fluorescence of HSA was calculated with the help of values of $I_{||}$ and $I_{\perp}$ in maximum of emission spectrum of protein fluorescence, where $I_{||}$ and $I_{\perp}$ – intensities of fluorescence, measured through a polarizer with axis directed parallel or perpendicular to polarization of exciting light. The obtained spectra were treated by the program FL Winlab (Perkin Elmer).

3. Results and Discussion

3.1. Non-Polarized Tryptophan Fluorescence of HSA in Investigations of Functional Transitions of HSA during Variation of pH at Absence of Surfactants

Proteins play the central role in realization and regulation of almost all biological processes taking place in organisms at molecular level, therefore the problem of interrelation of structure and function of protein macromolecules is one of central in a modern science. For effective work of proteins the certain stability of protein macromolecule, which is provided with complex system of bonds and interactions, is necessary. Protein macromolecules are capable to undergo structural rearrangements under the influence of various factors and agents. Two types of such dynamic rearrangements are possible: transition of protein from native state to denaturated functionally inactive state (denaturated transition) and transition between two functionally active states (functional transition). Changes in intramolecular dynamics of proteins in the solutions in absence of surfactants, occurring at change of pH of solutions in a range 3.5 - 6.0, belong to functional transitions, i.e. lie in limits of native protein structures. At first in this work the functional transitions of HSA at change of pH of solutions in absence of surfactants by research of fluorescent-spectral characteristics of amino-acidic residue of tryptophan in HSA molecule have been considered. The dependences of intensity I_{fl}^{max} (Figure 1, curve 1) and wavelength λ_{fl}^{max} (Figure 1, curve 2) in maximum of spectrum of tryptophan fluorescence of HSA on pH were received. It is seen (Figure 1, curve 1) that with increase of pH from 3.5 up to 6.0 there is increase of I_{fl}^{max}, caused by change of the environment of the residue of tryptophan in HSA molecule in process of small conformational rearrangements. Besides the increase of tryptophan fluorescence of HSA at increase of pH (Figure 1, curve 2) the red shift of spectrum of fluorescence is observed: λ_{fl}^{max} is shifted from 334.0 nm at pH 3.5 up to 349.8 nm at pH 6.0.

Variation of pH of solutions causes changes of ionization of protein groups, what leads to conformational functional changes in the protein in limits of native structure (in the specified range of values of pH). Conformational functional transitions in HSA, occurring within its native structure, change an environment of protein fluorophore – amino-acidic residue of tryptophan, and, hence, change a tryptophan fluorescence of HSA.

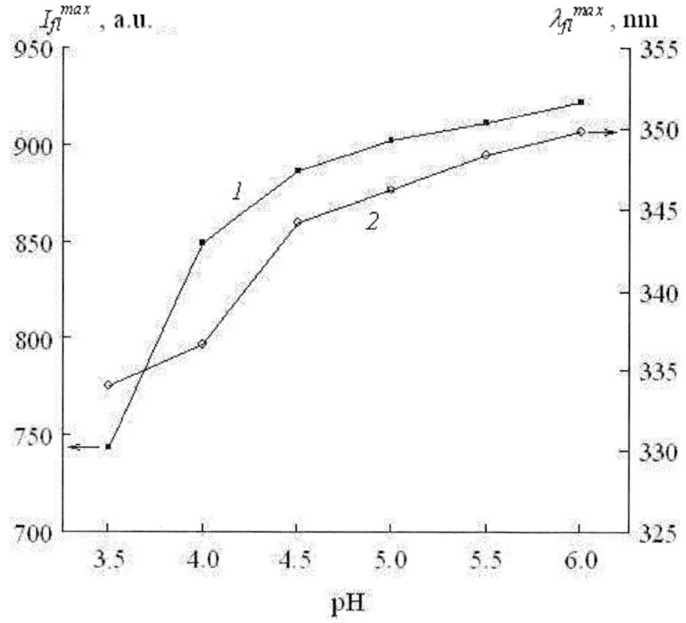

Figure 1. Dependences of intensity Iflmax (1) and wavelength □flmax (2) in maximum of spectrum of tryptophan fluorescence (λexc = 295 nm) of HSA (5 μM) on pH of solutions in absence of SDS and CTAB.

Thus, decrease of value of pH from 6.0 up to 3.5 leads to decrease of I_{fl}^{max} and to shift of λ_{fl}^{max} to short-wave region what is caused by conformational functional transition of protein (so-called N-F-transition). This N-F-transition of HSA and corresponding change of tryptophan protein fluorescence are explained by protonating of carboxyl groups of protein and are characteristic for all serum albumins [1].

3.2. Non-Polarized Tryptophan Fluorescence of HSA in Solutions of Ionic Surfactants SDS and CTAB

For an estimation of structural conformational condition of HSA molecules at denaturation under action of SDS the spectra of non-polarized tryptophan fluorescence of HSA in the solutions with various concentration of SDS (0 - 7 mM) at various values of pH (3.5 - 6.0) are investigated.

In Figure 2.*a* the dependences of intensity in maximum of spectra of tryptophan fluorescence of HSA (I_{fl}^{max}) on concentration of SDS at various values of pH are shown. In the solutions with SDS the tryptophan fluorescence of HSA is quenched: I_{fl}^{max} in solutions in the presence of SDS is smaller, than I_{fl}^{max} in the solutions without SDS. Quenching of tryptophan fluorescence of HSA in the presence of SDS speaks about denaturation owing to which, at unfolding of HSA globule, the chromophore group of tryptophan becomes more accessible to molecules of water, that quench this fluorescence.

From Figure 2.*a* it is seen that more strong quenching of tryptophan fluorescence of HSA in the presence of identical concentration of SDS is observed at lower values of pH. The following dependence of quenching of fluorescence of HSA in the solutions containing SDS on pH is found out: the higher value of pH – the smaller is the quenche of fluorescence of HSA.

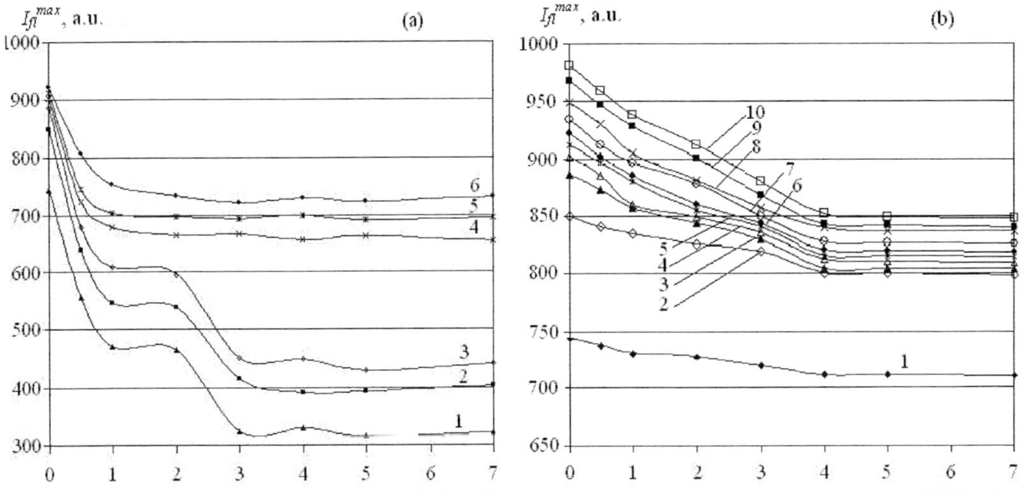

Figure 2. Dependences of intensity I_{fl}^{max} in maximum of spectrum of tryptophan fluorescence (λ_{exc} = 295 nm) of HSA (5 μM) on concentration of SDS (*a*) and on concentration of CTAB (*b*) at various values of pH: 3.5 (1), 4.0 (2), 4.5 (3), 5.0 (4), 5.5 (5), 6.0 (6), 6.5 (7), 7.0 (8), 7.5 (9), 8.0 (10).

This behavior one can explain in the main by electrostatic mechanism of interaction of HSA with SDS. Molecules of SDS in a solution dissociate into positively charged ions of sodium and dodecyl sulfate anions, and dodecyl sulfate anions interact with HSA. At values of pH, lower than pI of HSA, molecules of HSA, as a whole, are charged positively, therefore there is an intensive binding of positively charged macromolecules of HSA with dodecyl sulfate anions and hence strong denaturation of HSA, accompanying by the strong quenching of tryptophan fluorescence of HSA in solutions with SDS in comparison with the solutions without SDS is observed. With increase of pH the positive charge of macromolecules of HSA decreases, and at values of pH, higher than pI of HSA, molecules of HSA have, as a whole, a negative charge and consequently there is a weak binding of dodecyl sulfate anions with negatively charged molecules of HSA, through a few reminding positively charged sites. Consequently the weak denaturation of HSA accompanying with the weak quenching of tryptophan fluorescence of HSA is observed. Thus, stronger denaturation of protein under the action of SDS occurs at values of pH, lower than pI of HSA.

The non-linear dependences I_{fl}^{max} on concentration of SDS at various values of pH (Figure 2.*a*) one can explain by the complex multi-stage mechanism of denaturation of HSA under action of SDS, in dependence on whether higher or lower pI of HSA the value of pH is.

At values of pH 3.5 - 4.5, lower than pI of HSA, denaturation of HSA under action of SDS is not simple one-stage process, but is two-stage process (Figure 2.*a*). At concentration of SDS, smaller than 1 mM, the quenching of tryptophan fluorescence of HSA is observed, and in the range of concentration of SDS from 1 up to 2 mM the value of I_{fl}^{max} is almost constant. This is the first transitive stage of protein denaturation – decondensation of globules of HSA. At increase of SDS concentration to 3 mM the further quenching of tryptophan fluorescence of HSA is observed – this is the second stage of denaturation - full unfolding. At increase of SDS concentration from 3 up to 7 mM the I_{fl}^{max} varies slightly that specifies on full denaturation of HSA molecules. The further increase of concentration SDS does not change the given system.

The two-stage quenching of intrinsic fluorescence of HSA at increase of concentration SDS at values of pH, lower than pI of HSA, one can explain by two-stage mechanism of denaturation and consecutive conformational rearrangements of protein globule, leading to opening of tryptophan and to increase of its availability to the molecules of water quenching its fluorescence.

At values of pH 5.0 – 6.0, higher than pI of HSA, the process of denaturation of HSA under action of SDS passes only the first stage (Figure 2.*a*). At increase of concentration of SDS up to 1 – 2 mM the quenching of tryptophan fluorescence of HSA occurs, i.e. denaturated decondensation of protein globules is observed (the first stage of denaturation), leading to increase of availability of tryptophan of HSA for molecules of water quenching its fluorescence. The further increase of concentration of SDS (> 2 mM) at these values of pH does not result in the second stage of denaturation: I_{fl}^{max} remains almost constant.

Thus, unlike denaturation at values of pH, lower than pI of HSA, passing through two stage (decondensation and full unfolding), at values of pH, higher than pI of HSA, denaturation stops at the first stage – decondensation of protein globules (in investigated range of concentration of SDS).

We also investigated spectra of tryptophan fluorescence of HSA in solutions with various concentration of CTAB (0 – 7 mM) at various values of pH (3.5 – 8.0).

In Figure 2.*b* the dependences of intensity in maximum of spectrum of tryptophan fluorescence of HSA (I_{fl}^{max}) on concentration of CTAB at various values of pH are shown. At all values of pH in solutions with CTAB the quenching of tryptophan fluorescence of HSA (Fig. 2*b*) is observed. Quenching of fluorescence of HSA in the presence of CTAB in solutions speaks about denaturation of protein under action of CTAB – decondensation of HSA globules, opening of hydrophobic pocket with tryptophan and opening of tryptophan for water molecules quenching its fluorescence.

It is seen (Figure 2.*b*) that denaturation of HSA under action of CTAB at all investigated values of pH (3.5 – 8.0) has one-stage character – protein globules are decondensated gradually up to 4 mM of CTAB, the further increase of concentration of CTAB practically nothing changes in system.

The value of quenching of tryptophan fluorescence of HSA in solutions with CTAB depends on value of pH: at values of pH, lower than pI of HSA (4.7), quenching of fluorescence is insignificant, at values of pH, higher than pI of HSA, quenching of fluorescence is significant. The given fact one can explain, in the main, by electrostatic mechanism of interaction of HSA and CTAB. In the solution the molecules of CTAB dissociate into cethyltrimethylammonium-cations and bromine-anions. At values of pH, higher than pI of HSA (4.7), molecules of HSA as a whole are negatively charged, and cethyltrimethylammonium-cations intensively bind to protein, this leads to essential denaturation and to strong quenching of fluorescence of HSA. At pH, lower than pI of HSA, cethyltrimethylammonium-cations weakly bind to positively charged molecules of HSA, this leads to weak denaturation and to weak quenching of fluorescence of HSA.

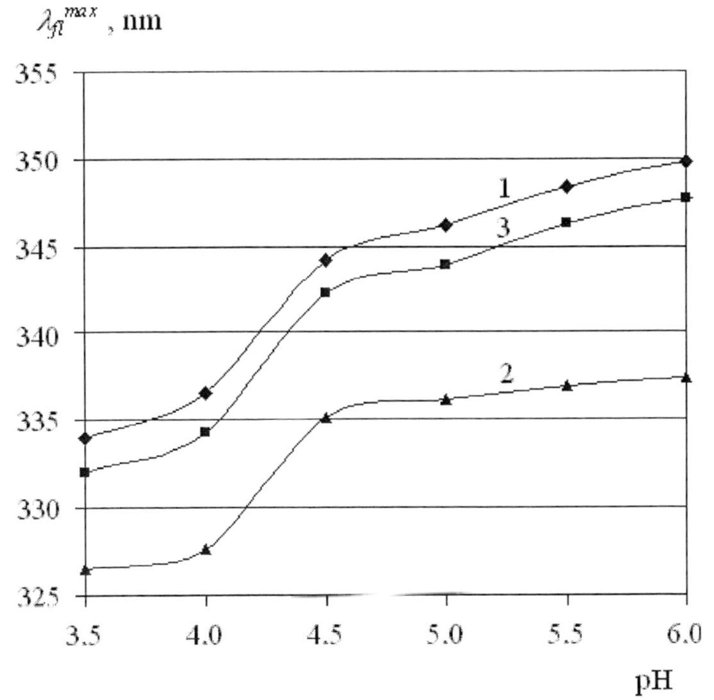

Figure 3. Dependences of wavelength λ_{fl}^{max} in maximum of spectrum of tryptophan fluorescence (λ_{exc} = 295 nm) of HSA (5 μM) on values of pH of solutions: without surfactants (1), with 0.5 mM of SDS (2), with 0.5 mM of CTAB (3).

The mechanism of denaturation of HSA under the action of ionic surfactants (SDS and CTAB) is investigated also by the analysis of position of wavelength of maximum of spectrum of tryptophan fluorescence of HSA (λ_{fl}^{max}). In Figure 3 dependences of λ_{fl}^{max} on values of pH of solutions, as without surfactants, so with 0.5 mM of SDS and 0.5 mM of CTAB are presented. It is necessary to note that at increase of pH the value of λ_{fl}^{max} shifts to the large wavelengths as for the solutions with surfactants, so for the solutions without surfactants.

At addition in a solution of 0.5 mM of SDS the sharp blue shift of λ_{fl}^{max} occurs, and at addition of 0.5 mM of CTAB this blue shift is rather small (Figure 3).

This blue shift of λ_{fl}^{max} in solutions with surfactants one can explain by the change of the nearest environment of chromophore group of tryptophan of HSA as consequence of rearrangements of protein globule under influences of the surface-active ions of surfactants.

One can see that the changes of position of λ_{fl}^{max} are sensitive only to changes of the nearest environment of tryptophan and consequently do not reflect of stages of denaturation of HSA. But changes of I_{fl}^{max} reflect both local rearrangements of the nearest environment of tryptophan, and more peripheral changes of globule of HSA.

3.3. Polarized Tryptophan Fluorescence of HSA in Solutions of Ionic Surfactants SDS and CTAB

In this work the investigations of polarized tryptophan fluorescence of HSA in solutions with ionic surfactants at various values of pH were done.

As it is known, changes of polarization of fluorescence are caused by two reasons – firstly, by rotational diffusion of fluorophores and, secondly, by non-irradiation transfer of energy between fluorophores. Thanks to selection of experimental conditions (strongly diluted solutions of protein (5 μM) are investigated) the contribution from the second reason – non-irradiation transfer of energy between fluorophores – is absent. Thus, only rotational diffusion of fluorophore – tryptophan in protein molecule – influences on polarization of fluorescence of HSA at these experimental conditions.

This polarization of fluorescence of tryptophan residue of HSA molecule is, generally speaking, caused by rotation of whole molecule of protein, by rotation of the domain II of protein, containing tryptophan, and by rotation of tryptophan relative nearest environment. The steady-state measurements of polarized fluorescence of HSA allow one to analyze the rotation of the whole molecule of protein, and the contributions of rotation of the domain, containing tryptophan, and of rotation of tryptophan nearest environment in this work are considered as small.

The dependences of degree of polarization (*P*) of tryptophan fluorescence of HSA on concentration of SDS (Figure 4.*a*) at various values of pH are obtained. The degree of polarization *P* of tryptophan fluorescence of HSA is calculated by values of $I_{||}$ and $I_{\perp}$ in maximum of emission spectrum of HSA fluorescence.

It is seen from Figure 4.*a*, that the values of *P* increase up to 1 mM of SDS concentration for all values of pH – this is the first stage of denaturation of HSA – decondensation of protein globules. The further behavior of *P* strongly depends on values of pH.

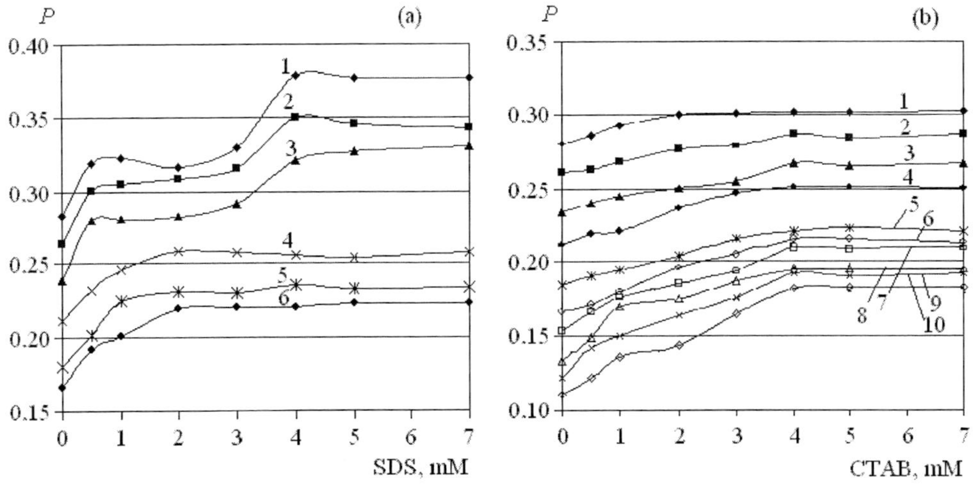

Figure 4. Dependences of degree of polarization (*P*) of tryptophan fluorescence (λ_{exc} = 295 nm) of HSA (5 μM) on concentration of SDS (*a*) and on concentration of CTAB (*b*) at various values of pH: 3.5 (1), 4.0 (2), 4.5 (3), 5.0 (4), 5.5 (5), 6.0 (6), 6.5 (7), 7.0 (8), 7.5 (9), 8.0 (10).

At pH, higher than isoelectric point of HSA pI (4.7), the further increase (more than 1 mM) of concentration of SDS practically does not change values of *P* (Figure 1.a) – this is the one-stage denaturation.

At pH, lower than pI of HSA, other character of dependences of *P* on concentration of SDS is observed (Figure 4.*a*): in the range of SDS concentration from 1 mM up to 2 mM the value of *P* is almost constant, in the range of SDS concentration from 2 mM up to 4 mM there is a further increase of *P*. This behavior one can explain by increase of the linearly-longitudinal sizes of HSA molecules at unfolding of amino-acidic chain. This is the second stage of denaturation of HSA – a stage of full unfolding of amino-acidic chain. At further increase in SDS concentration over 4 mM (up to 7 mM) values of *P* are almost constant. Full denaturation of HSA molecules and full unfolding of chain of HSA occur.

Hence, by two-stage increase in values of *P* at increase of SDS concentration it is possible to conclude that at pH, lower than pI of HSA, denaturation of HSA in the presence of SDS represents two-stage process, and at pH, higher than pI of HSA, denaturation of HSA has only one stage.

It is seen that larger increase of *P* with increase of concentration of SDS in HSA solutions takes place at values of pH, lower than pI of HSA.

Also the dependences of degree of polarization (*P*) of tryptophan fluorescence of HSA on concentration of CTAB (Figure 4.*b*) at various values of pH are obtained. The degree of polarization *P* of tryptophan fluorescence of HSA is calculated by values of $I_{||}$ and $I_{\perp}$ in maximum of emission spectrum of HSA fluorescence.

As it is seen from Figure 4.*b*, the values of *P* increase in range up to 4 mM of CTAB for all values of pH that specifies on decondensation of protein globules and on increase of the linearly-longitudinal sizes of HSA molecules at partial unfolding of amino-acidic chain. The further increase (larger than 4 mM) of CTAB concentration practically does not change values of *P*. It is seen that larger increase of *P* with increase of concentration of CTAB in HSA solutions takes place at values of pH, higher than pI of HSA.

3.4. Rotational Diffusion of HSA Molecules in Solutions with Ionic Surfactants SDS and CTAB

The method of the polarized fluorescence allows one to estimate parameters of rotational diffusion of fluorophores. The quantitative theory of rotational depolarization has been offered by F. Perren in the model of rotational diffusion. The expression for degree of polarization P of fluorescence, received on the basis of this theory, is:

$$\frac{1}{P} = \frac{1}{P_0} + \left(\frac{1}{P_0} - \frac{1}{3}\right) \cdot \frac{kT\tau_0}{V\eta},$$

where T – absolute temperature, η – viscosity of solution, V – volume, k – constant Boltzmann, τ_0 – average time of quenching of fluorescence of fluorophore (for tryptophan of HSA this is 2.8 ns), P_0 – limiting degree of polarization of fluorescence. Thus, by changing viscosity of solutions (by addition of various concentration of sucrose) and postponing $1/P$ on axis of ordinates, and T/η on axis of abscissae, we receive a straight line, which cuts on an axis of ordinates a segment equal to $1/P_0$. Tangent of angle φ of a slope of this straight line to an axis of abscissae,

$$tg\varphi = \left(\frac{1}{P_0} - \frac{1}{3}\right) \cdot \frac{k\tau_0}{V},$$

for known value τ_0 allows one to determine a size of molecular volume

$$V = \frac{(3 - P_0) \cdot k \cdot \tau_0}{3 \cdot P_0 \cdot tg\varphi}$$

and, hence, Einstein's effective hydrodynamic radius a

$$a = \sqrt[3]{\frac{3V}{4\pi}}.$$

Using this data, it is possible to determine time of a rotational relaxation (or disordering owing to thermal diffusion) ξ of fluorophore by the formula:

$$\xi = \frac{V\eta}{Tk},$$

where V – molecular volume.

For fluorophores it is possible also to determine a coefficient of rotational diffusion D_{rot}:

$$D_{rot} = \frac{kT}{6\eta V} = \frac{1}{6\xi}.$$

By a variation of viscosity of solutions by addition of various concentration of sucrose the time of rotational relaxation, coefficient of rotational diffusion and Einstein's effective radius of HSA molecules in solutions with various concentrations of SDS and CTAB at various values of pH are determinated. In Figure 5.*a* the dependences of coefficient of rotational diffusion D_{rot} of HSA molecules on concentration of SDS at various values of pH are presented. It is seen that more strong decrease of D_{rot} of HSA molecules in solutions with SDS takes place at values of pH, lower than pI of HSA, that indicates deep and strong denaturation. Also it is seen that sharp decrease of D_{rot} of HSA molecules occurs at concentration of SDS, lower than 0.5 mM, at all values of pH that indicates the change of geometrical configuration of HSA globules – increase of the linearly-longitudinal sizes of HSA molecules at its decondensation in the first stage of denaturation. The further increase of SDS concentration leads to rather small one-stage decrease of D_{rot} of HSA molecules at values of pH, higher than pI of HSA, and to rather large two-stage decrease of D_{rot} of HSA molecules at values of pH, lower than pI of HSA. In Figure 5.*b* the dependences of coefficient of rotational diffusion D_{rot} of HSA molecules on concentration of CTAB at various values of pH are presented. In solutions with CTAB at all values of pH there is a decrease of values of D_{rot} of HSA molecules, explained by denaturation of HSA under action of CTAB and corresponding decondensation of protein globules (increase of linearly-longitudinal sizes) of HSA. It is seen that more strong decrease of D_{rot} of HSA molecules in solutions with CTAB (up to 4 mM of CTAB) occurs at values of pH, higher than pI of HSA, what indicates deep and strong denaturation. The dependences of time of rotational relaxation ξ, or time of disordering owing to thermal diffusion, of HSA molecules on concentration of SDS (Figure 6.*a*) and on concentration of CTAB (Figure 6.*b*) at various values of pH are determinated. It is registered that at all values of pH in solutions with SDS and CTAB the value of ξ of HSA molecules is essential more than time of life of fluorophore – tryptophan residue in HSA (2.8 ns) what causes high polarization of fluorescence of solutions of HSA with surfactants.

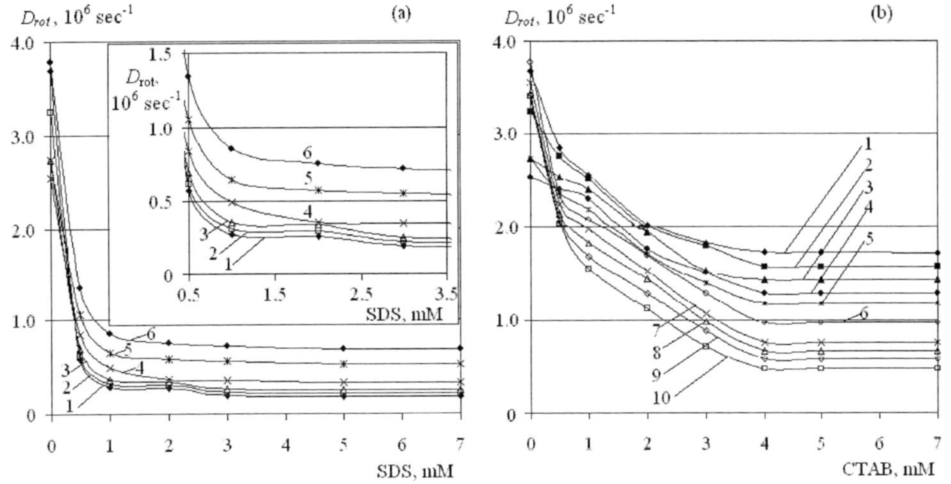

Figure 5. Dependences of coefficient of rotational diffusion D_{rot} of HSA molecules on concentration of SDS (*a*) and on concentration of CTAB (*b*) at various values of pH: 3.5 (1), 4.0 (2), 4.5 (3), 5.0 (4), 5.5 (5), 6.0 (6), 6.5 (7), 7.0 (8), 7.5 (9), 8.0 (10).

It is seen (Figure 6) that at increase of concentration of SDS and CTAB in solutions there is an increase of ξ of HSA molecules, and the size of this increase of ξ of HSA molecules is determinated by value of pH: in solutions with SDS a more essential increase of ξ occurs at values of pH, lower than pI of HSA, whereas in solutions with CTAB a more essential increase of ξ takes place at values of pH, higher than pI of HSA.

The dependences of Einstein's effective radius a of HSA molecules on concentration of SDS (Figure 7.*a*) and on concentration of CTAB (Figure 7.*b*) in solutions at various values of pH are presented.

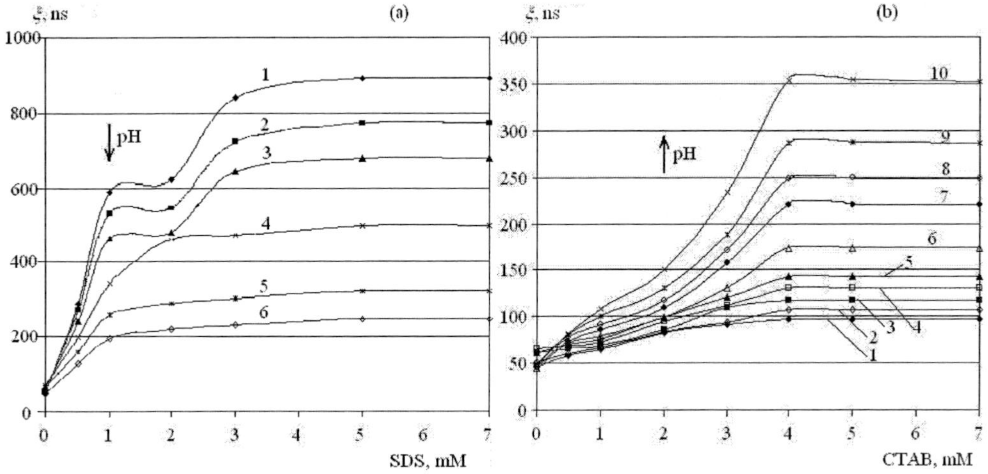

Figure 6. Dependences of time of rotational relaxation ξ of HSA molecules on concentration of SDS (*a*) and on concentration of CTAB (*b*) at various values of pH: 3.5 (1), 4.0 (2), 4.5 (3), 5.0 (4), 5.5 (5), 6.0 (6), 6.5 (7), 7.0 (8), 7.5 (9), 8.0 (10).

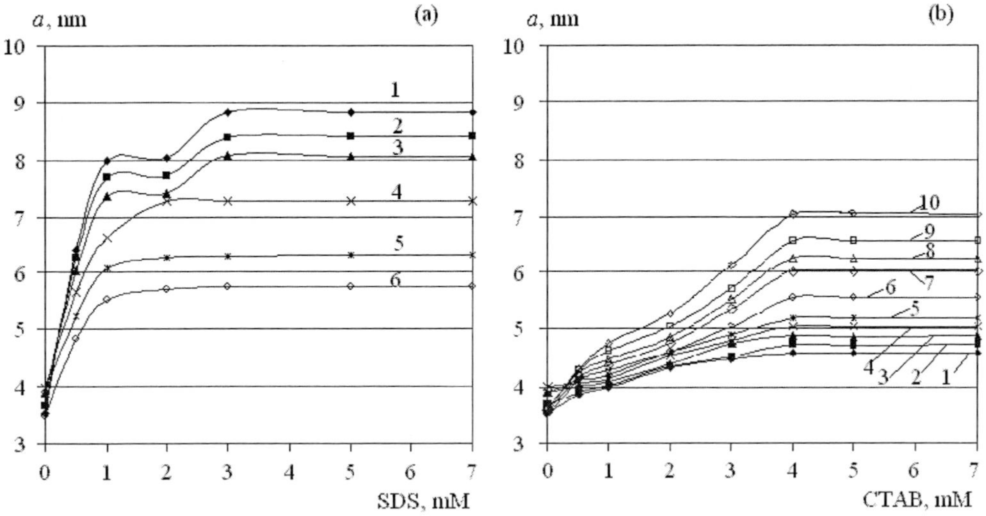

Figure 7. Dependences of Einstein's effective radius a of HSA molecules on concentration of SDS (*a*) and on concentration of CTAB (*b*) in solutions at various values of pH: 3.5 (1), 4.0 (2), 4.5 (3), 5.0 (4), 5.5 (5), 6.0 (6), 6.5 (7), 7.0 (8), 7.5 (9), 8.0 (10).

It is known that in the base of the model of rotational depolarization by Perren lie the following conditions – isotropic distribution of molecules, dipole character of its radiation, hydrodynamic description of Brownian motion of molecules. Thus, the radius*a* of HSA molecules, determinated in spherical hydrodynamic approach, reflects not the real geometrical size of HSA molecules, which at passage of denaturation under the action of SDS and CTAB get more and more extended, non-spherical geometrical form, but radius *a* shows the effective size of HSA molecules convenient for estimation of degree of depth of denaturation of protein under action of SDS and CTAB.

It is seen (Figure 7) that more strong increase in the sizes of HSA molecules in solutions with SDS takes plarece at values of pH, lower than pI of HSA, what indicates more deep denaturation of protein. With increase of concentration of SDS at values of pH, higher than pI of HSA, the increase of *a* of HSA molecules has one-stage character, but at values of pH, lower than pI of HSA, the increase of *a* has two-stage character.

It is seen (Figure 4.b) that more strong increase of the sizes of HSA molecules in solutions with CTAB takes place at values of pH, higher than pI of HSA, what indicates more deep denaturation of protein.

CONCLUSION

The tryptophan fluorescence of human serum albumin (HSA) at addition of ionic surfactants (anionic surfactant sodium dodecyl sulfate SDS and cationic surfactant cethyltrimethylammonium bromide CTAB) in protein solution at different values of pH was investigated, what gave information about mechanism of denaturation of HSA under action of these ionic surfactants.

In this work were investigated as functional transitions of HSA (within it native structures), occurring at change of pH of solutions in absence of surfactants, so denaturated transitions of HSA occurring under action of SDS and CTAB at various values of pH.

Character of quenching of tryptophan fluorescence of HSA in solutions with ionic surfactants gives the information on mechanisms of denaturation of HSA under the action of these surfactants at various values of pH.

The two-stage quenching of tryptophan fluorescence of HSA at increase of concentration of SDS specifies to two-stage character of denaturation of HSA: the first stage – decondensation of protein globules (up to 1 – 2 mM SDS), the second stage – full unfolding of amino-acidic chain of protein (3 – 4 mM SDS). At values of pH, lower than pI of HSA, denaturation passes through both stages. At values of pH, higher than pI of HSA, denaturation stops at the first stage and the increase of concentration of SDS changes nothing in system.

By analysis of quenching of non-polarized tryptophan fluorescence of HSA at increase of concentration of CTAB it is revealed that denaturation of HSA under action of cationic surfactant CTAB at all investigated values of pH has one-stage character, unlike two-stage denaturation of HSA under action of anionic surfactant SDS that specifies in rather deeper denaturation of HSA under action of anionic surfactants in comparison with cationic surfactants.

The mechanism of denaturation of HSA under the action of ionic surfactants also is determinated by research of polarized tryptophan fluorescence of HSA, and by calculation of parameters of rotational diffusion of molecules of HSA in solutions with surfactants.

By analysis of values of degree of polarization of fluorescence of HSA, of time of rotational relaxation, of coefficient of rotational diffusion and of Einstein's effective radius of molecules of HSA in solutions with various concentration of SDS and CTAB at various values of pH the conclusion about one-stage denaturation of HSA under action of cationic CTAB and complex denaturation of HSA under action of anionic SDS (at values of pH, higher than pI of HSA, there is one-stage denaturation, but at values of pH, lower than pI of HSA, there is two-stage denaturation) is made.

Thus by the analysis of tryptophan fluorescence of HSA and by the analysis of parameters of rotational diffusion of molecules of HSA in solutions the following conclusions are made: more effective and deep denaturation of HSA under the action of SDS occurs at values of pH, lower than pI of HSA, and more deep denaturation of HSA under the action of CTAB occurs at values of pH, higher than pI of HSA, that speaks in favor of electrostatic interactions.

REFERENCES

[1] Peters, T. All about Albumin. New York: Academic Press; 1996.

[2] Dawson, R., Elliot, D., Elliot, W., Jones, K. Data for Biochemical Research. Oxford: Clarendon Press; 1986.

[3] Jackson, M. Molecular and Cellular Biophysics. Cambridge: Cambridge University Press; 2006.

[4] Moriyama, Y., Ohta, D., Hachiya, K., Mitsui, Y., Takeda, K. Fluorescence behavior of tryptophan residues of bovine and human serum albumins in ionic surfactant solutions: a comparative study of the two and one tryptophans of bovine and human albumins. *Journal Protein Chemistry*, 1996 v. 15, p. 265-272.

[5] Lissi, E., Abuin, E., Lanio, M.E., Alvarez, C. A new and simple procedure for the evaluation of the association of surfactants to proteins. *Journal Biochemical Biophysical Methods*, 2002 v. 50, p. 261-268.

[6] Gelamo, E.L., Silva, C.H.T.P., Imasato, H., Tabak, M. Interaction of bovine (BSA) and human (HSA) serum albumins with ionic surfactants: spectroscopy and modeling. *Biochemical Biophysical Acta*, 2002 v. 1594, p. 84-99.

[7] Dockal, M., Carter, D.C., Ruker, F. Conformational transitions of the three recombinant domains of human serum albumin depending on pH. *Journal Biological Chemistry*, 2000 v. 275, p. 3042-3050.

[8] Santos, A., Duarte, A.G., Fedorov, A., Martinho, J.M.G., Moura, I. Rubredoxin mutant A51C unfolding dynamics: a Forster resonance energy transfer study. *Biophysical Chemistry*, 2010 v. 148, p. 113-137.

[9] Mukherjee, S., Saha, B., Das, A.K. Differential chemical and termal unfolding pattern of Rv3588c and Rv1284 of Mycobacterium tuberculosis – a comparison by fluorescence and circular dichroism spectroscopy. *Biophysical Chemistry*, 2009 v. 141, p. 94-104.

[10] Baranov, A.N., Vlasova, I.M., Mikrin, V.E., Saletsky, A.M. Investigation of denaturation of serum albumin by laser correlation spectroscopy method of dynamic light scattering. *Journal Applied Spectroscopy*, 2004 v. 71, p. 911-915.

[11] Vlasova, I.M., Zemlyansky, A.Yu., Saletsky, A.M. The spectral-luminescence characteristics of eosin in human serum albumin solutions at its denaturation induced by sodium dodecyl sulfate. *Journal Applied Spectroscopy*, 2006 v. 73, p. 743-747.

[12] Vlasova, I.M., Polyansky, D.V., Saletsky, A.M. Raman spectroscopy in investigations of mechanism of human serum albumin denaturation under action of sodium dodecyl sulfate. *Laser Physics Letters*, 2007 v. 4, p. 890-894.

[13] Vlasova, I.M., Saletsky, A.M. Fluorescence of tryptophan in the denaturation of human serum albumin under the action of sodium dodecyl sulfate. *Russian Journal Physical Chemistry B*, 2009 v. 3, p. 976-980.

[14] Vlasova, I.M., Saletsky, A.M. Investigation into denaturation of human serum albumin by sodium dodecyl sulfate through albumin intrinsic fluorescence. *Journal Applied Spectroscopy*, 2009 v. 76, p. 536-541.

[15] Vlasova, I.M., Saletsky, A.M. Investigation of denaturation of human serum albumin under action of cethyltrimethylammonium bromide by Raman spectroscopy. *Laser Physics*, 2011 v. 21, p. 239-244.

[16] Vlasova, I.M., Vlasov, A.A., Saletsky, A.M. Interaction of ionic detergent cethyltrimethylammonium bromide with human serum albumin at various values of pH: spectroscopic study. *Journal Molecular Structure,* 2010 v. 984, p. 332-338.

In: Serum Albumin: Structure, Functions and Health Impact ISBN: 978-1-62100-231-4
Editors: R. J. Alekseev and A. L. Rebane

Chapter 6

Albumin in Drug Delivery

Giuliano Siligardi and Rohanah Hussain*
Diamond Light Source, Science Division, Harwell Science and Innovation Campus, Chilton, United Kingdom

Abstract

Albumin is the most abundant protein in human plasma, being present at a concentration of 30-50 g/l. It has several important functions in the blood including assistance in maintaining osmotic pressure; transport of hormones (in particular fat soluble ones); transportation of fatty acids to the liver; transportation of drugs; and maintenance of pH. It has a long plasma half life – typically 20 days (Peters 1996). This combination of low biological activity, long half life and ability to bind fatty (and therefore poorly aqueous soluble) molecules makes albumin an attractive candidate for incorporation into drug delivery/formulation systems and its use in this role has been examined over the last twenty years (Peters 1996). More recently there has also been a growing awareness that albumin may, under certain circumstances, be selectively accumulated by solid tumours (Clorius et al, 1995; Goldshaid et al; 2010). Clearly this accumulation of albumin offers the potential for improved delivery of drugs to specific sites of action, particularly to tumours. The search for effective drug delivery systems is one of the major challenges facing pharmaceutical research, especially for biomedically important molecules such as proteins, peptide-based vaccines, tumour therapeutic agents, antimicrobials and lipodrugs. A procedure has been developed whereby human serum albumin (HSA) can be use as a delivery vehicle for a number of these biological molecules by exploiting its physiological role as the bodies' main fatty acid carrier. Using essentially fatty acid free HSA (HSAff) it is possible to form stable complexes with compounds that contain alkyl chains (called lipo-compounds). Two lipo-compounds have been used to develop this system, a novel antimicrobial peptide and the neurotransmitter γ-amino-n-butyric acid GABA conjugated with C8 or C14 alkyl chains (Hussain and Siligardi 2006, 2010). Both lipo-compounds were evaluated confirming that the formation of HSA-lipo compound complexes had a mutual stabilizing effect on both HSAff and lipo-compounds. The protease enzymes pronase was used to show that the alkyl chains of the lipo-compounds bound to HSAff conferred a similar if not greater

*E-mail: rohanah.hussain@diamond.ac.uk

resistance to enzymatic degradation than the HSA for clinical use such as Baxter Albumin and Zenalbumin, which contain sodium caprylate and acetyl tryptophanate. Here we indicated that the use of HSAff as a carrier for lipidated drugs might confer higher biostability to the lipidated drugs providing a novel formulation method for therapeutic use. The increased stability of the lipo-compounds when formulated using the HSAff was not observed when HSA containing fatty acid (HSAfa) was used (Hussain and Siligardi 2006 and 2010). Furthermore in the case of the antimicrobial lipopeptide there was an increased in activity with the HSAff formulation suggesting that besides conferring stability it also enhanced bioavailability of compounds that would otherwise exist as insoluble micelles in aqueous media. These findings have allowed us to develop a simple and effective way of delivering lipo containing compounds using fatty acid free HSA as the drug carrier.

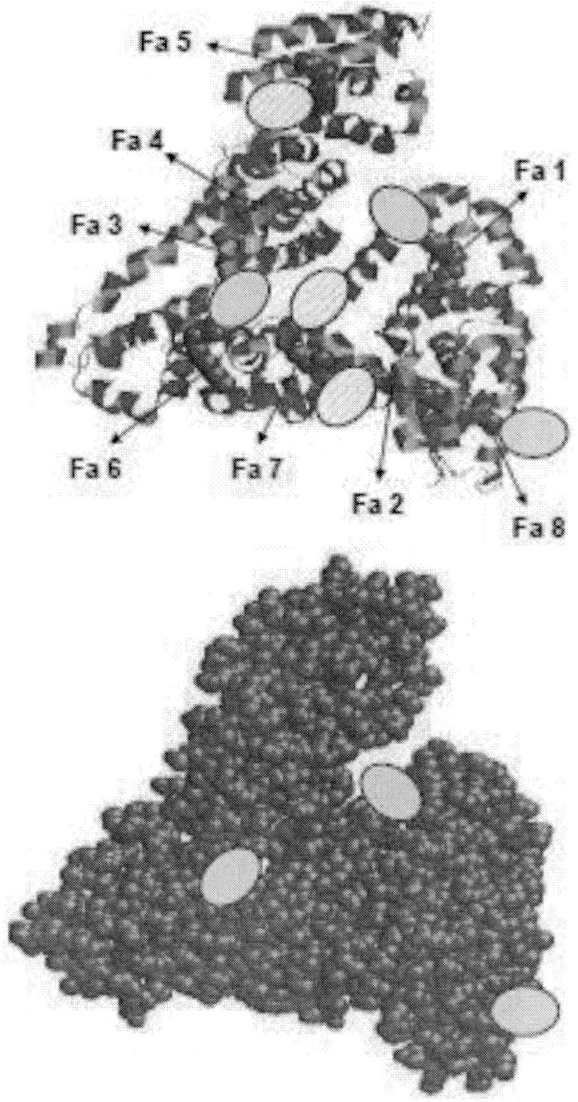

Figure 1. Cartoon representation of HSA (green) complexed with lipo-drugs. FAs are the fatty acid binding sites. Yellow circle (solid front view, striped back view) represents drug coupled to fatty acid (red).

INTRODUCTION

Pharmacokinetics, bioavailability and interactions of pharmaceuticals are important features for the drug formulation and dosage determination. The drug delivery system can crucially influence these pharmaceutical properties which are vital for the drug therapeutic and/or prophylactic action. Numerous drug delivery systems are currently being developed with various degrees of success and applicability (Scherrmann, 2002). Biological molecules such as proteins, peptide vaccines, peptide-base tumour therapeutic agents, and peptide-base antimicrobials have particular problems such as susceptibility to endogenous proteases and distribution to target sites. The use of lipidic moieties covalently attached to such molecules has been used to improve absorption and transportation *in vivo* (Hussain, 1992). However this strategy has met with limited success. Biostability to enzymatic degradation still poses a problem with the peptide-base drugs containing lipidic moieties. To counteract this problem an increased number of lipidic moieties have to be covalently-linked to these drugs which poses another formulation problem i.e. solubility for *in vivo* administration. This will limit the amount that can be administered into the body, hence affecting its efficacy.

In this chapter we present the use of an exogenous preparation of essentially fatty-acid free albumin with lipiadted drugs as a novel carrier vehicle (Figure 1). A procedure whereby bioactive compounds tagged with C8 and C14 alkly chains but not only can be formulated with exogenous essentially fatty acid-free human serum albumin (HSAff) will be discussed.

MATERIAL AND METHODS

HSAff and HSAfa were obtained from Sigma, Baxter HSA was obtained from Baxter Healthcare Ltd and Pronase® Protease, Nuclease free from *Streptomyces* griseus was obtained from Calbiochem. Delipidised Baxter was prepared using dialysis. The lipo-Gaba, GabaC8 and GabaC14 were synthesised using crown ether chemistry (Hussain, 1992). The lipopeptide RH01 as synthesised using standard Fmoc/TFA solid phase peptide synthesis. The UV and circular dichroism (CD) data were collected with a Jasco spectropolarimeter J720 with time constant 4s, bandwidth 1nm, using a 0.05cm pathlength cell (Hellma) and Diamond B23 beamline end-station B with ring current 200mA, 0.28mm slitwidth equivalent to 0.8nm bandwidth, scan speed 38nm/min and using 0.02cm pathlength cell (Hellma).

Formulation of HSAff with lipo-compounds. The lipo-Gaba compounds were prepared in ethanol, lipopeptide RH01 (myristoyl-FARKGALRQ) in aqueous solutions and HSAff added to give the required molar ratios. The mixtures were incubated with gentle agitation.

GABase studies. The GABase assays for GABA was preformed using the method described by Jakoby (1962) with the modification that esterase (70units) was added for the assay of lipo-Gaba, GabaC8 and GabaC14. The GABase assay monitors the reduction of NADP to NADPH spectroscopically at 340nm, pH 8.6 at 25°C, as a function of time using GABA as a substrate.

Pronase studies. The CD signals were monitored at 220nm as a function of time after pronase addition (1/100 w/w). The rate of albumin degradation in the presence of lipo-compounds were then monitored. The percentage of pronase stability was calculated by dividing the CD data of the formulation with pronase by the CD data without pronase and multiplied by 100.

S aureus time kill studies. Lipopeptide RH01 time-kill assays were preformed on *Staphylococcus aureus* NCTC 6571 Oxford strain (Colindale, UK) in suspension medium (PBS) using standard microbiological techniques (Hussain and Siligardi 2010).

DISCUSSION

Several examples are discussed in terms of formulation, stabilization, solubility and efficacy.

Formulation of HSA with Lipo-Compound

The full potential of HSA as a drug delivery system can only be achieved if it is formulated exogenously with the lipo-compounds concerned. We have developed methods to fully load lipo-compounds exogenously into HSAff and to assess the stability of the formulation to enzymes and temperature degradations. The *in vitro* data show that the formulation of delipidised Baxter HSA (DL Bax) with lipopeptide RH01, molar ratio (1:2) is better stabilised by up to 50% when pre-incubated 1 hour before pronase addition compared to the non pre-incubated formulation (Figure 2). This exogenous use of HSAff as a novel drug delivery system is supported by the fact that fatty acids require time to fully bind to defatted albumin (Peters, 1996). These observations are also consistent with *in vivo* data reported by Lee *et al*, (1991) on an antimicrobial lipopeptide daptomycin (N-dodecyl cyclic peptide) where the concentration of total and free lipo-peptide in six human subjects was reduced by 90% within the first hour after intravenous injection. The increased stability in the first hour of drug injection is very im[portant as the majority of druf elimination occurs during this time (ref?).

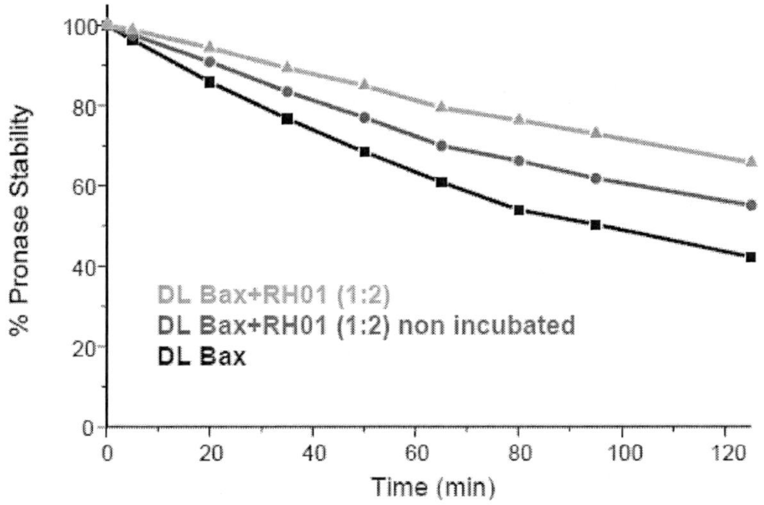

Figure 2. Effect of preincubation to the pronase stability of delipidised Baxter HSA with RH01 (1:2).

Stabilization of Lipo-Gaba by HSAff

The GabaC8 stability was assessed using the GABase assay and pronase susceptibility. There was no GABase activity with GabaC8 as the substrate (data not shown). Only with the addition of plasma esterase to the assay mixture GabaC8 became susceptible to GABase (Figure 3). Formulations of GabaC8 with both HSAfa and HSAff showed reduced GabaC8 susceptibility to GABase (Figure 3). However, the formulation of GabaC8 with HSAff showed a remarkable resistance to esterase hence to GABase (Figure 3) 10 fold higher than using the HSAfa. These results suggest that the tagged GabaC8 is protected from esterase degradation as it is bound tightly to HSAff as opposed to HSAfa, which contains approximately 4moles of fatty acid per mole of albumin.

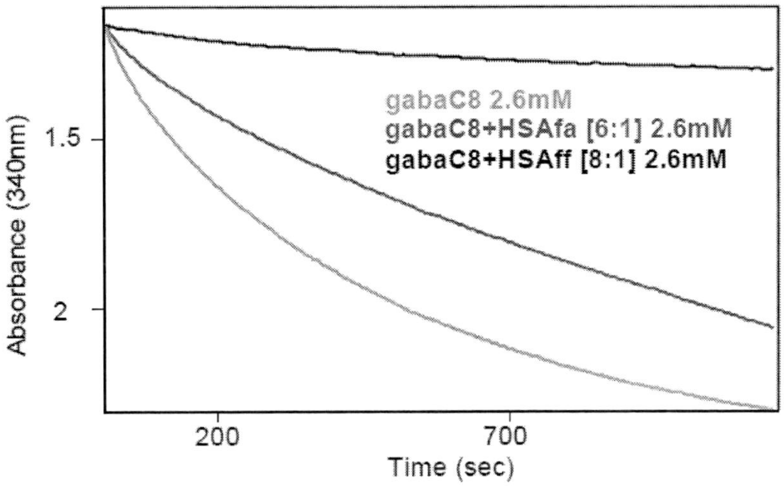

Figure 3. Lipo-Gaba stability to GABase with and without HSAfa and HSAff.

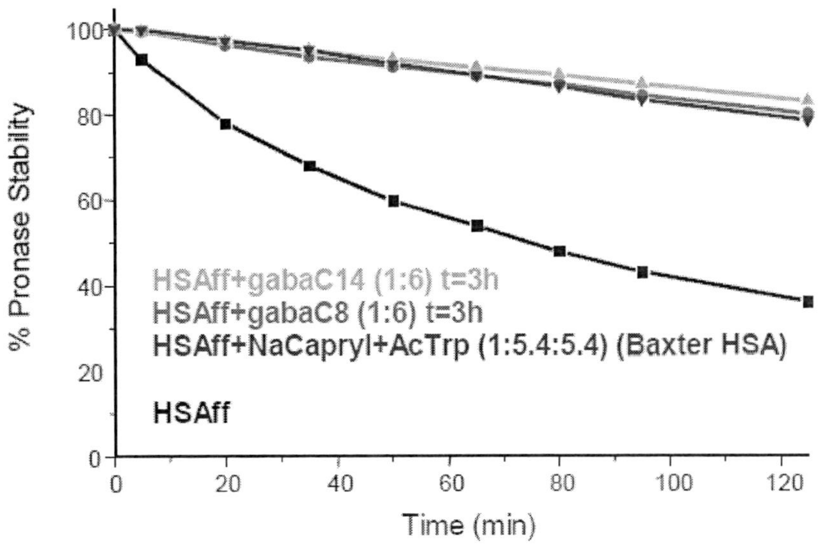

Figure 4. Pronase stability of HSAff with and without lipo-Gaba compounds compared to Baxter HSA.

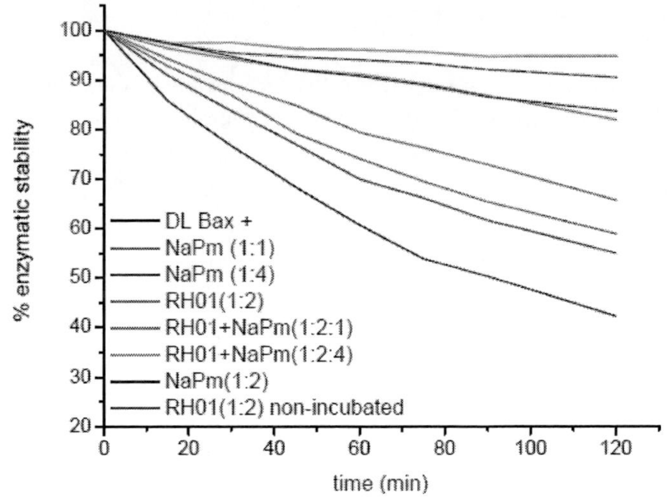

Figure 5. Stability of DL Bax HSA to pronase 1/100w/w degradation in the presence of Na Palmitate and RH01.

Stabilization of HSAff by Lipo-Compounds

Interestingly, not only does HSAff enhance the stability of lipo-compounds to enzymatic biodegradation, but the lipo-compounds themselves in turn stabilises HSAff from protease degradation (figures 4 and 5). The result show that the stability of defatted albumin containing the FDA recommended stabilisers Na caprylate and N-acetyl tryptophanate in the molar ratio 1:5.4:5.4 (Baxter HSA) is also achieved by the addition of GabaC8 or GabaC14 in the molar ratio 1:6 (figures 4 and 5) and lipopetide RH01 1:2 (Hussain and Siligardi, 2010). For these formulations similar effects were also observed for thermal stability assays at 60°C for 10 hours (data not shown). This is the pastorisation process that albumin from plasma has to undergo to inactivate pathogenic viruses (Peters, 1996).

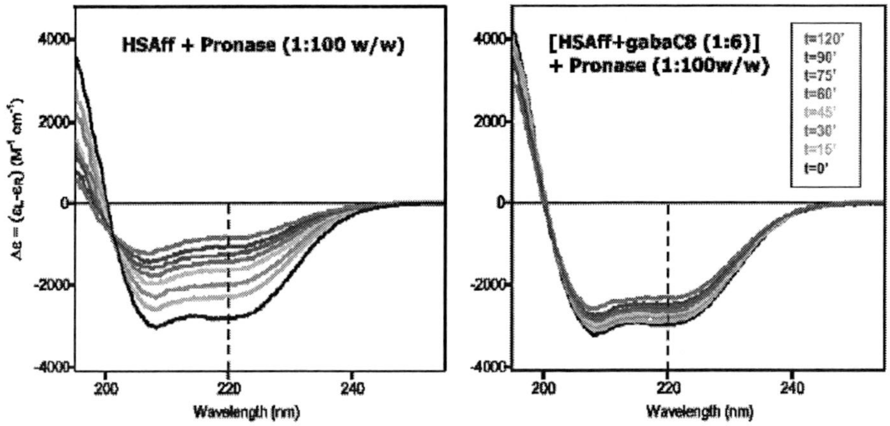

Figure 6. Pronase enzymatic degradation of HSAff and lipidated molecule bound to HSAff at 37°C as a function of time monitored by CD spectroscopy.

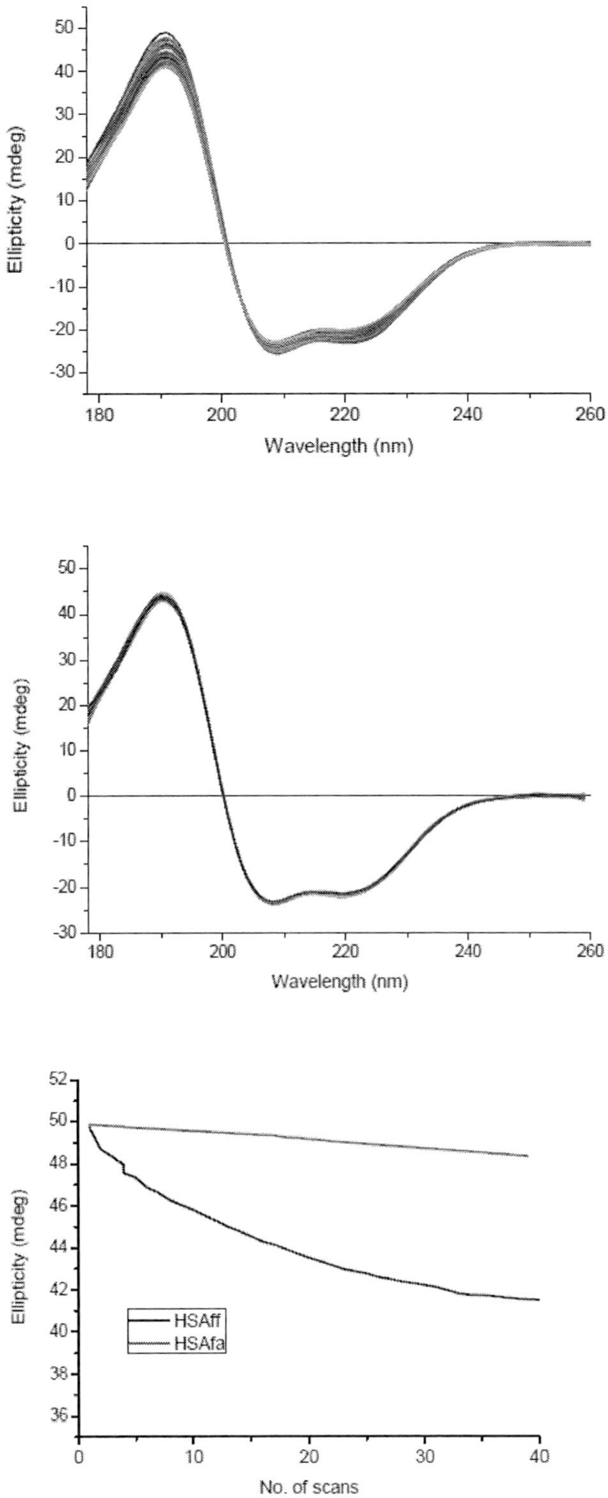

Figure 7. Comparasion of HSAff (top) and HSA with fatty acid (bottom) stability to high flux UV, B23 beamline, 200mA ring current as function of multiple scans (100 scans).

These results were consistent with the stabilizing effect of lipidated compounds on albumin such as Na caprylate (Na octanoate) in the molar ratio 1:5.4 (Baxter HSA) and GabaC8 or GabaC14 in the molar ratio 1:6 (Hussain and Siligardi, 2006) (Figure 6), sodium palmitate (NaPm) and antimicrobial lipopeptide (Hussain and Siligardi, 2010).

This stabilization effect of lipocompounds bound to HSAff can also be assayed using high photon flux far-UV irradiation monitoring the changes in secondary structure of the HSAff of the drug formulations as a function of time. This was achieved using Diamond B23 circular dichroism beamline (www.diamond/B23) end-station module B.. This is illustrated in figure 7 where the highly collimated light beam of B23 beamline allows the monitoring of the denaturation process of HSAff with and without fatty acid (figure 7) as a function of repeated scans. These results indicate the enhanced stability effect of lipo-molecules when bound to HSAff, which support the use of this type of formulation as a delivery system

Solubility of Lipo-GABA

HSAff enhances the solubility to lipophilic compounds by binding to hydrophobic moieties of lipo-drugs . This facilitates dissolution of poorly water soluble compounds such as lipoGABA, GABA-C14 (figure 8). By visual inspection in figure 8 the solution of gabaC14 with aquous HSAff appears transparent whilst the gabaC14 in aquoues NaCl 0.9% is clearly a milky emulsion. This is consistent with the light scattering of the gabaC14 emulsion revealed by its UV spectrum (figure 8).

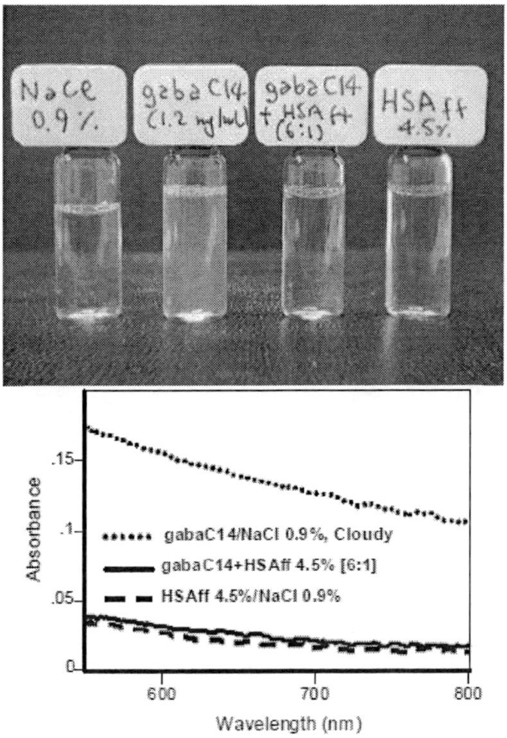

Figure 8. (top) HSAff showing enhanced solubility to GABA.C14 (1.2mg/ml) and (bottom) shows high absorbance due to light scattering.

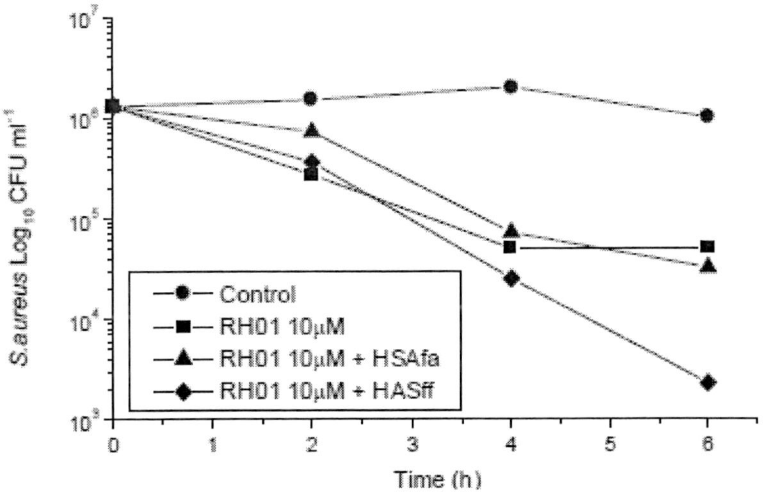

Figure 9. Time kill curves of RH01 formulations on *S. aureus*. RH01 formulations was added to washed cells of *S. aureus* corresponding to 10^6 cells ml^{-1} in PBS and the effect on viability determined at timed intervals as CFU ml^{-1} and compared to that for control cells. Each datum is the mean of at least three experiments and each experiment was carried out in triplicate. For each datum the SEM was less than 10% therefore error bars were excluded for clarity.

Efficacy of HSAff-Antimicrobial Lipopeptide RH01 Complex

Another property of human serum albumin in the fatty acid-free form (HSAff) when used as an exogenous material in a drug-formulation is that it can confer increased efficacy to the carried lipo-drug. We have found that the HSAff enhanced the antimicrobial activity of a lipopeptide RH01 against *S aureus* (table 1). The activity of RH01 formulated with HSAff was twice as potent when compared to the lipopeptide alone or with HSA containing bound fatty acid (HSAfa) (Hussain and Siligardi 2006, 2010). RH01 formulated with HSAff had a faster and greater rate of kill towards S *aureus,* Figure 9. The difference in potency widens more significantly when samples are subjected to appropriate enzymatic degradation conditions (table 2). This is consistent with the protective effect of HSAff on the lipopeptide towards digestive enzymes in the body. The results demonstrate that HSAff can be used as an external ingredient to enhance the biological activities of other lipo-drugs by regulating their biostability. This exogenous use of HSAff as a novel drug delivery system is supported by the fact that fatty acids require time to fully bind to defatted albumin (Peters, 1996). These observations are also consistent with *in vivo* data reported by Lee *et al*, (1991) on an antimicrobial lipopeptide daptomycin (N-dodecyl cyclic peptide) where the concentration of total and free lipo-peptide in six human subjects was reduced by 90% within the first hour after intravenous injection.

CONCLUSION

In this chapter we clearly demonstrated the potential use of HSAff in the formulation of lipo-tagged phamaceuticals that would otherwise have a limited use. HSAff provides a compelling case for its use as an exogenous ingredient in drug delivery technology. Hence, the application of HSAff formulations has a number of important benefits over other delivery systems, such as compatibility with host as it is a naturally occurring protein. HSAff can be used in sustained delivery of lipo-drugs via its depot effect through equilibrium with endogenous fatty acids and the real possibility of reduced dosage of the lipo-drugs due to increased stability thus extending *in-vivo* half-life of the drug and reducing drug toxicity. HSAff can also regulate the biodistribution of these lipo-drugs via increased penetration index, thus enabling the crossing of membrane barriers (Makriyannis et al 2005). Another potential benefit of HSAff in formulation is the ability to prolong the shelf-life of the lipo-drug via mutual stabilization. In drug discovery stage, HSAff provides a route to reduce the need to increase the lipid component of the drug.

All these factors are especially vital for patient compliance and crucial for drugs that have narrow therapeutic index hence improving patient's quality of life.

Table 1. HSAff lowers the MIC of antimicrobial lipopeptide RH01 towards S. aureus and E. coli. † Each datum is the mean of at least three experiments and each experiment was carried out in triplicate

Samples	MIC (μM)	
	E coli	S.aureus
RH01+HSAff (6:1)	12	1.6
RH01+HSAfa (6:1)	23.8	3.2
RH01+Baxter HSA (6:1)	49.8	3.2
RH01	23.8	3.2

Table 2. Lipopeptide RH01 was stabilised against proteolytic enzymes using HSAff towards *S.aureus*

Samples + Pronase 1/250 w/w	MIC (mg/ml) S.aureus
RH01+ HSAff (6:1)	0.12
RH01+HSAfa (6:1)	0.5
RH01	0.5

REFERENCES

Clorius JH, Sinn, H, Manke HG, Schrenk HH, Blatter, J, Werling C, Friedrich EA, Voges J, Bahner M, Sturm V; "Serum albumin (SA) accumulation by bronchogenic tumours: a tracer technique may help with patient selection for SA-delivered chemotherapy" *Eur. J. Nucl. Med,* 1995, 22 (9): 989-96.

Goldshaid L, Rubinstein E, Brandis A, Segal D, Leshem, N, Brenner, O, Kalchenko V, Eren D, Yecheskel T, Salitra Y, Salomon Y, Scherz A, "Novel design principles enable specific targeting of imaging and therapeutic agents to necrotic domains in breast tumors", *Breast cancer Research,* 2010, 12:R29.

Hussain R. "Synthesis and structural elucidation of novel highly lipophilic CNS and antiviral drugs" *PhD thesis*, University of London, 1992.

Hussain R and Siligardi G: Fat-free Albumin as a Novel Drug Delivery System *International Journal of Peptide Research and Therapeutics* 2006; 12(3): 311–315.

Hussain R and Siligardi G: Novel Drug Delivery System for Lipophilic Therapeutics of Small Molecule, Peptide-based and Protein drugs 2010; *Chirality* 22: E44-E46.

Jakoby, W.B Methods in Enzymology 1962, V, 771-774.

Kaparissides C, Alexandridou S, Kotti K and Chaitidou S: Recent advances in novel drug delivery systems. *Journal of Nanotechnology Online* 2006; 2:1-11.

Lee B L, Sachdeva M and Chambers H F. "Effect of protein binding of daptomycin on MIC and antibacterial activity" *Antimicrobial Agents and Chemotherapy* 1991, 35, 2505-2508.

Makriyannis A, Guo J and Tian X: Albumin enhances the diffusion of lipophilic drugs into the membrane. *Life Sciences* 2005; 77: 1605-1611.

Peters T, All about Albumin, *Academic Press*, 1996.

Scherrmann, J.-M. "Drug delivery to brain via the blood-brain barrier" *Vascular Pharmacology* 2002, 38, 349-354.

Wunder A, Muller-Ladner U, Stelzer, EHK, Funk J, Neumann E, Stehle G, Pap T, Sinn, H, Gay S and Fiehn C,. "Albumin-based drug delivery as Novel Therapeutic Approach for Rheumatoid Arthritis" *J. Immunology,* 2003, 170, 4793-4801.

In: Serum Albumin: Structure, Functions and Health Impact ISBN: 978-1-62100-231-4
Editors: R. J. Alekseev and A. L. Rebane

Chapter 7

INFLUENCE OF EXOGENOUS AND ENDOGENOUS IONS ON THE PROPERTIES OF BSA

D. Giacomazza[1*], M. R. Mangione[1*], D. Bulone[1], V. Martorana[1], G. Navarra[2] and P. L. San Biagio[1]

[1]Consiglio Nazionale delle Ricerche, Istituto di Biofisica, Palermo, (Italy)
[2]Università di Palermo, Dipartimento di Fisica, Palermo, (Italy)

ABSTRACT

The relation between several pathological diseases (Alzheimer, BSE, Creutzfeldt-Jacob disease, etc.) and the formation of proteinaceous deposits in plaques, amyloid fibrils and filaments has led a great deal of renewed attention to the topic of protein aggregation. Different factors such as pH, temperature, solvents, protein concentration, cosolutes, etc., modulate the aggregation process. In particular, the presence of metal ions can modify inter- or intra-molecular interaction thus exerting different effects on proteins stability.

In the present chapter we show that the addition of exogenous ions to a solution of partially denaturated Bovine Serum Albumin (BSA) promotes molecular aggregation and gel formation (cold gelation). On the other hand, we describe how BSA native structure is stabilized by the presence of endogenous ions, which are so strongly bound that can be separated by HPLC treatment only.

INTRODUCTION

The stabilization of proteins is of paramount importance in many fields ranging from basic and medical biochemistry, food science (Ratnaparkhi, G.S. and Varadarajan R., 2001; Ragoonanan and Aksan, 2007) and pharmaceutical technology (Brange et al., 1992). In the recent years much interest has been focused on the proteins aggregation (Dobson, 2004) and particularly, on the interaction with metal ions. In fact, electrostatic interactions between side

[*] The two authors have contributed equally to the present work.

chains on the proteins surface can contribute to the stability: ions can interact with charged groups, and, in the case of multivalent ions, they can link different residues thus contributing to stabilize the native state (Gibson, 1996, McLean et al., 2002). On the other hand, ions can bind to the peptide bond because of its large dipole moment and destabilize the native state. In general, the destabilization occurs if ions bind more effectively to non-native than native protein states (MacLean et al., 2002).

In the last few years, an increased interest of the scientific community was directed to the role of deficiencies or excesses of metal ions in neurodegenerative syndromes. An example is Manganism, a disease common among manganese miner workers. The disease causes a brain damage due to the inhalation of manganese rich dust (Donaldson, 1987). The interaction with copper is responsible for the pathological aggregation of alpha-synuclein, a member of the family of the proteins linked to Parkinson's disease (PD) (Rasia et al., 2005; Davies et al., 2011), although it seems that the non-pathological form of alpha-synuclein binds both copper and iron ions to exert its ferrireductase enzymatic action (Davies et al., 2011). The familial amyotrophic lateral sclerosis is strictly linked to a gene encoding a cytosolic, Cu/Zn-binding, superoxide dismutase (SOD1), a homodimeric metalloenzyme that catalyzes the dismutation of the toxic superoxide anion O^-_2 to O_2 and H_2O_2 (Fridovich, 1986; Rosen et al., 1993). Wilson's (Tanzi et al., 93) and Menkes' diseases (Vulpe et al., 1993) are the two first diseases conclusively linked to altered copper metabolism. The prion protein (PrP), responsible of the Creutzfeldt-Jacob disease (CJD) is also widely known as a copper binding protein, being this linkage necessary for its normal cellular function. It was also suggested that the prion protein binds other metals, and among these, manganese. Recent data have shown that manganese can stabilize prions in the environment and that chelation therapy (linked to manganese) can extend the lifetime of animals affected by prion disease (Brown, 2011). In addition, the presence of Zn^{2+} or Cu^{2+} decreases the thickness of the synthetic fragment PrP106-126 fibrils, as observed by atomic force microscopy, and reduces its neurotoxicity on primary cultured rat hippocampal neurons (Kawahara et al. 2011). In the case of Alzheimer' disease (AD), the Amyloid-beta peptide (Abeta) forms amyloid plaques that are primary hallmarks of the disease. Increasing evidence demonstrates that some biometals, Zn^{2+} and Cu^{2+}, interact with Abeta, being zinc more effective than copper (Comai et al. 2003). They also have an influence on Abeta fibrillization and toxicity. Zinc and copper ions are abundantly present in the synaptic areas of the brain, and it is likely that their age-related dyshomeostasis is associated with AD pathology (Tougu et al., 2011).

It has been proposed that the metal ions can bind the Abeta peptide in two distinct ways, generically termed inter- and intra-molecular modes (Curtain et al. 2001). In the inter-molecular mode, Abeta molecules are supposed to be cross-linked throught "Abeta-metal-Abeta" bridges, whereas in the intra-molecular mode the atoms participating in the metal coordination belong to the same peptide (Curtain et al. 2001). Structural models for each of the two binding modes have been suggested in which different numbers of histidine residues are involved in the metal coordination. Thus, metal ions can act as inhibitors or promoters of protein aggregation depending on their concentration and binding mechanism (Navarra et al., 2007; Navarra et al., 2009a and 2009b). The addition of metal ions to the protein solution can affect the protein conformation and tendency to aggregation up to induce gel formation (Haque and Aryana, 2002; Navarra et al., 2009a and 2009b; Remondetto and Subirade, 2003).

In the present chapter we present some results on the destabilizing/stabilizing effect of endogenous or exogenous ions on Bovine Serum Albumin (BSA). Firstly, we show that the addition of exogenous metals promotes the gelation of partially denatured BSA molecules (cold gelation). The rheological properties of the final gel can be finely tuned by ion's type and concentration. In the second part of the chapter we describe the stabilizing effects of endogenous metal ions on BSA native structure. In fact, we show that the protein deprived of its endogenous ions through a HPLC treatment is less stable against thermal denaturation and aggregation.

1. Bovine Serum Albumin

BSA is one of the most studied macromolecules as protein model in several scientific fields (Carter and Ho, 1994). It is the major constituent of the proteinaceous plasma fraction (60%) and accounts for the 80% of the osmotic blood pressure (Barreca et al., 2010). With a molecular mass of 66 kDa, BSA is constituted by 583 amino acids (Hirayama et al., 1990). The secondary structure consists of 67% alpha helix, 23% extended chain and 10% turn. Seventeen disulphide bridges contribute to the BSA native conformation and no beta structures are present in the natively folded BSA (Carter and Ho, 1994; Weijers, 1977). Its isoelectric point is around 5. The tertiary structure consists of three globular domains, each of them containing two subdomains (Carter and Ho, 1994; Ostojic et al., 2007). The Serum Albumin structures are well preserved in mammalians (Kosa et al., 1997; Stewart et al., 2003) and a great analogy (67%) exists between BSA and Human Serum Albumin (He and Carter, 1992; Huang et al., 2004). Due to the presence of different binding regions, it is capable of binding a wide number of molecules such as bilirubin, fatty acids, drugs and hormones (Barreca et al., 2010) and, in general, substances that are otherwise insoluble in plasma. In particular, serum albumins (SA) are the main carrier of the plasmatic zinc (9-14 μM, 75-85%) and other several divalent ions, either essential or toxic such as Co^{2+}, Cu^{2+}, Cd^{2+} and Ni^{2+} (Lu et al., 2008), from the bloodstream to the requiring organs and cells. The uptake and delivery mechanisms are still unclear (Lu et al., 2008) but recent studies suggest a role of Fe^{+3} specific binding site (Xu et al., 2008). Although many details are still missing, four metal sites have been found in Serum Albumins (Lu et al., 2008):

1. the ATCUN (N-terminal copper and nickel-binding) site at the N-terminus of the polypeptidic chain, with an high specificity for copper and nickel;
2. the A-site, specific for Zn but capable of linking other divalent ions;
3. the B-site, with high affinity for Cd ions with unknown location;
4. the thiol of the Cys residue in position 34, appointed for gold and platinum ions.

The ATCUN motif is the most studied metal binding site on Albumins and it is present in different proteins. It requires the presence of a histidine in position 3 in the primary sequence.

The main site for Zn binding, A-site, has been identified in human SA (Stewart et al., 2003). It involves the His^{67} and His^{247} residues and lies at the interface of domains I and II. Two additional potential ligands, Asn^{99}, from domain I, and Asp^{249}, from domain II, are situated nearby. Spectroscopic and binding data on Dog Serum Albumin (Sarkar and Wigfield, 1968; Lau and Sarkar, 1971; Ryall, 1974) suggest the occurrence of a histidine-metal-albumin ternary complex although its existence has not been unambiguously determined. Available X-ray and ^{111}Cd NMR data indicate that the presence of fatty acids disrupts the binding between Zn ions and Site A (Peters, 1995). The competition for the A-site is suggested by the observation of an increased level of plasmatic zinc during conditions of increased free fatty acid mobilization, as it occurs after strenuous exercise (Volpe, et al. 2007).

The thiol group of the Cys^{34} residue is important because it is able to bind many drugs and, among these the anticancer drugs containing Pt (Kratochwil et al., 1999).

Recently a specific site for Fe^{3+} ion has been found in BSA. Although no free Fe^{2+} is present because all iron is bound to transferrin in a redox-inactive Fe^{3+} form, BSA provides a temporary sink for excess iron, thus protecting against its toxic effect (Xu et al. 2008).

Living organisms require varying amounts of heavy metals, and homeostatic processes maintain their concentration. Particularly, Cu, Zn and Fe, are of undisputed importance for the vital process taking place in cells and organs.

Copper, like iron, is frequently encountered in reactions involving dioxygen. The copper enzyme laccase catalyzes the oxidation of uroshiol (substance found in poison oak and ivy) in the production of Japanese lacquer giving to the material remarkable properties (Crichton, 2008).

Zinc, in addition to its use as a Lewis acid in enzyme catalysis, plays a structural role in stabilizing protein molecules. It is also involved in a characteristic motif, termed zinc finger, in a number of eukaryotic DNA-binding proteins (that regulate the transcription of DNA into RNA), as described by Aaron Klug (for a review see Klug A., 2010).

Iron is essential for almost all living organisms, most probably because of its role in forming the amino acid radicals required for the conversion of ribonucleotides to deoxyribonucleotides in the Fe-dependent ribonucleotide reductases (Crichton, 2008) and in oxygen transport.

2. The Effect of Exogenous Ions: BSA Cold Gelation

Based on the protein-ion interaction, the so-called "cold-gelation" process is one of the most recent methods to obtain gels starting from a concentrated protein solution (Hongsprabhas and Barbut 1997; Remondetto et al., 2002; Remondetto and Subirade, 2003). The process requires two experimental steps: a thermal treatment of the protein solution, at low ionic strength and below the denaturation temperature, and the addition of ions (Barbut and Foegeding, 1993) or pH lowering (Alting et al., 2004) after cooling the solution at room temperature. In this way the protein activation step is uncoupled from the subsequent gel formation. This alternative method to obtain protein gels has important applications in food technology where the protein gelation is generally induced by heating. The latter has three main disadvantages: i) the non-optimal use of the food protein content because not all the molecules form aggregates and contribute to the final gel; ii) the difficulty of predicting the final texture, iii) the degradation of heath-labile flavors (Alting, 2003). Cold gelation is also valuable in pharmaceutical and medical industries and, in particular, in tissue engineering because the gel formation does not need high temperatures incompatible with the cell life.

2.1. Thermal Treatment of BSA Solution

To study the effect of different ions on the cold gelation of BSA, the protein was initially incubated for two hours at 58 °C (Navarra et al. 2009a), that is below the denaturation threshold (67°C).

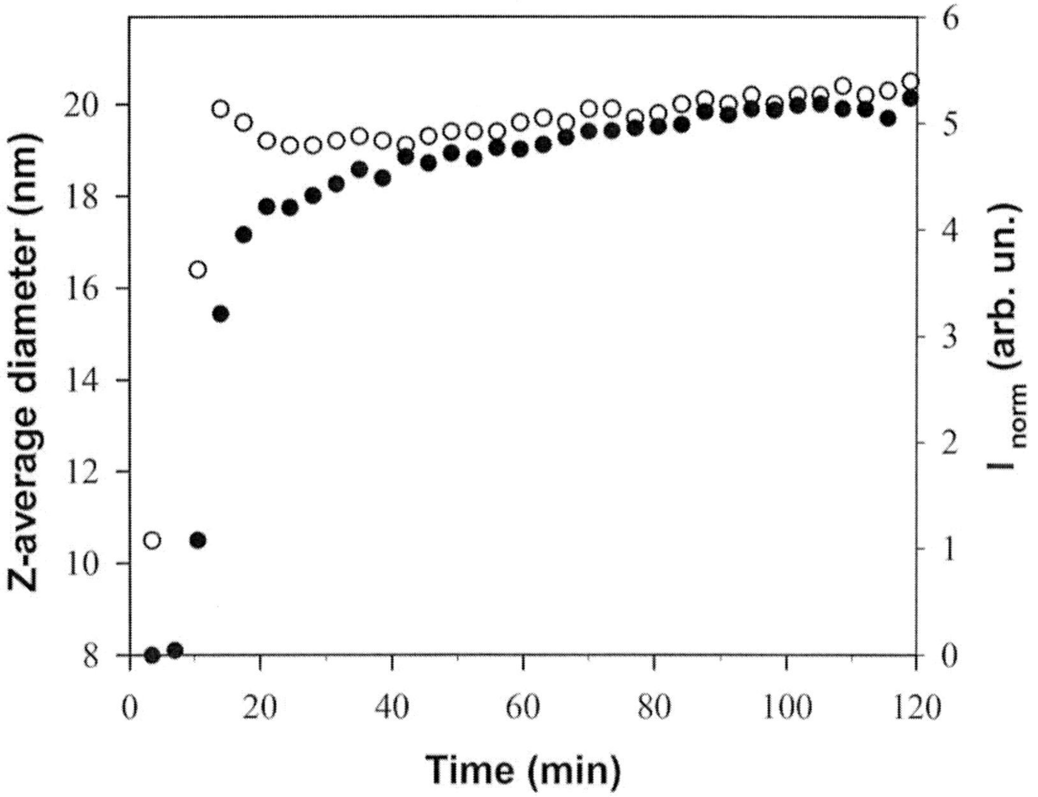

Figure 1. Time course of the average diameter (empty circles) and normalized light scattered intensity (black circles) of a sample of 1mM BSA (pH = 7) incubated at T = 58 °C.

After 20 minutes from incubation, BSA forms small aggregates. Figure 1 shows the increase of the normalized light scattered intensity and mean Z-averaged diameter of the species in solution. Figure 2 shows the size distribution, by number (A) and intensity (B), at initial (t_0), intermediate (t_i) and final (t_f) times. We note that, even after two hours of incubation, the aggregates present in solution are still small, and their dimension does not change up to 8 hours (data not shown).

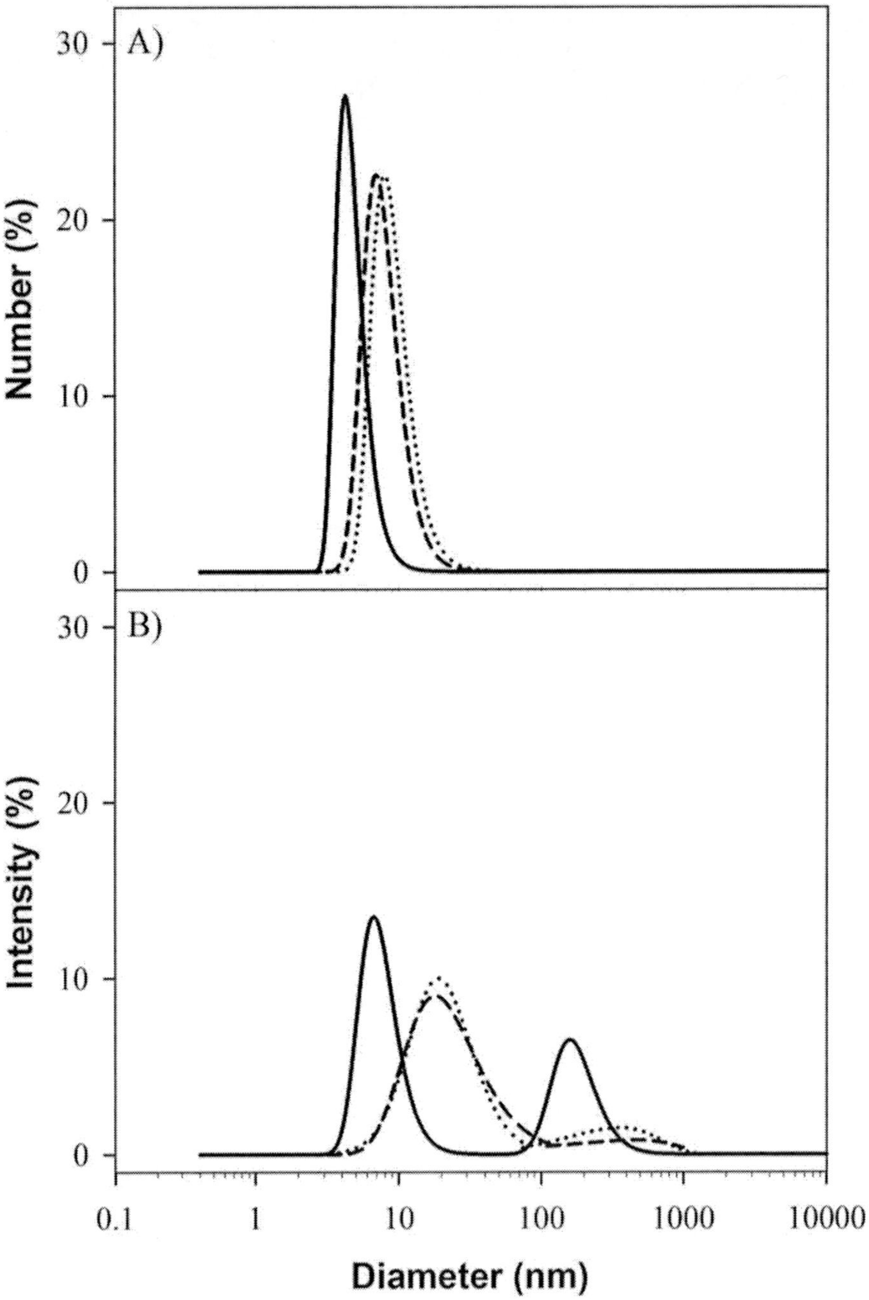

Figure 2. Number (panel A) and intensity (panel B) average size distribution of aggregates at different stages of the kinetics at T = 58 °C: t = 7 min (solid line), t = 20 min (dashed line) and t = 120 min (dotted line).

To follow the BSA tertiary and secondary structure changes, the IR absorption spectra of Amide II and Amide I bands were recorded during the incubation. The Amide II band is primarily due to the N—H in plane bending and it is sensitive to change of tertiary structure. Indeed, the isotopic substitution of hydrogen, ^{1}H, with deuterium, ^{2}H, inside the protein, caused by a partial opening of the protein, shifts the Amide II band towards lower wavenumbers (Amide II' band) (Kavanagh et al., 2000). The Amide I band is attributed to an out of phase combination of C=O and C-N stretching of amide groups (Bakker et al. 2005; Dong et al., 1990) and its location and shape are sensitive to the secondary structure of the protein (Byler and Susi, 1986; Surewicz and Mantsch H.H., 1988).

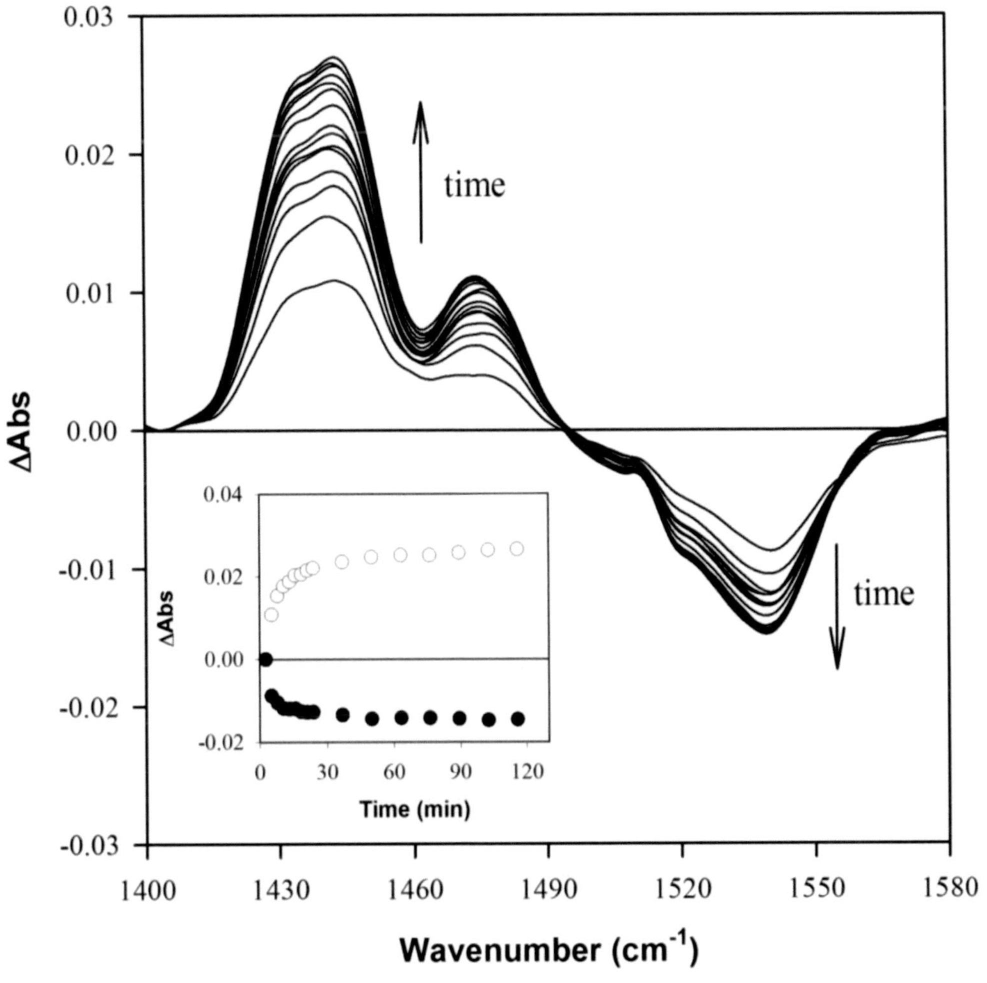

Figure 3. IR difference absorption spectra of Amide II and Amide II' bands measured on a sample of 1mM BSA (pH = 7) at different stages of the 2-hours incubation at T = 58 °C. The inset shows the intensity value of Amide II' (empty circles) and Amide II (full circles) bands, recorded at 1442 cm^{-1} and 1540 cm^{-1} respectively.

Figure 3 shows the IR absorption difference spectra measured at different time during the incubation of a BSA solution at 58 °C. Data show a decrease of the Amide II band (1510 – 1580 cm^{-1}) and the simultaneous increase of Amide II' band. The inset shows the time evolution of Amide II peak (1540 cm^{-1}) compared with the Amide II' peak (1442 cm^{-1}). The two signals reach the plateau in about 20 min in agreement with the light scattered intensity shown in Figure 1. Figure 4A shows the absorption spectra in the region of Amide I band, measured at the beginning and the end of the incubation. A structural change is observed after 2 hrs.

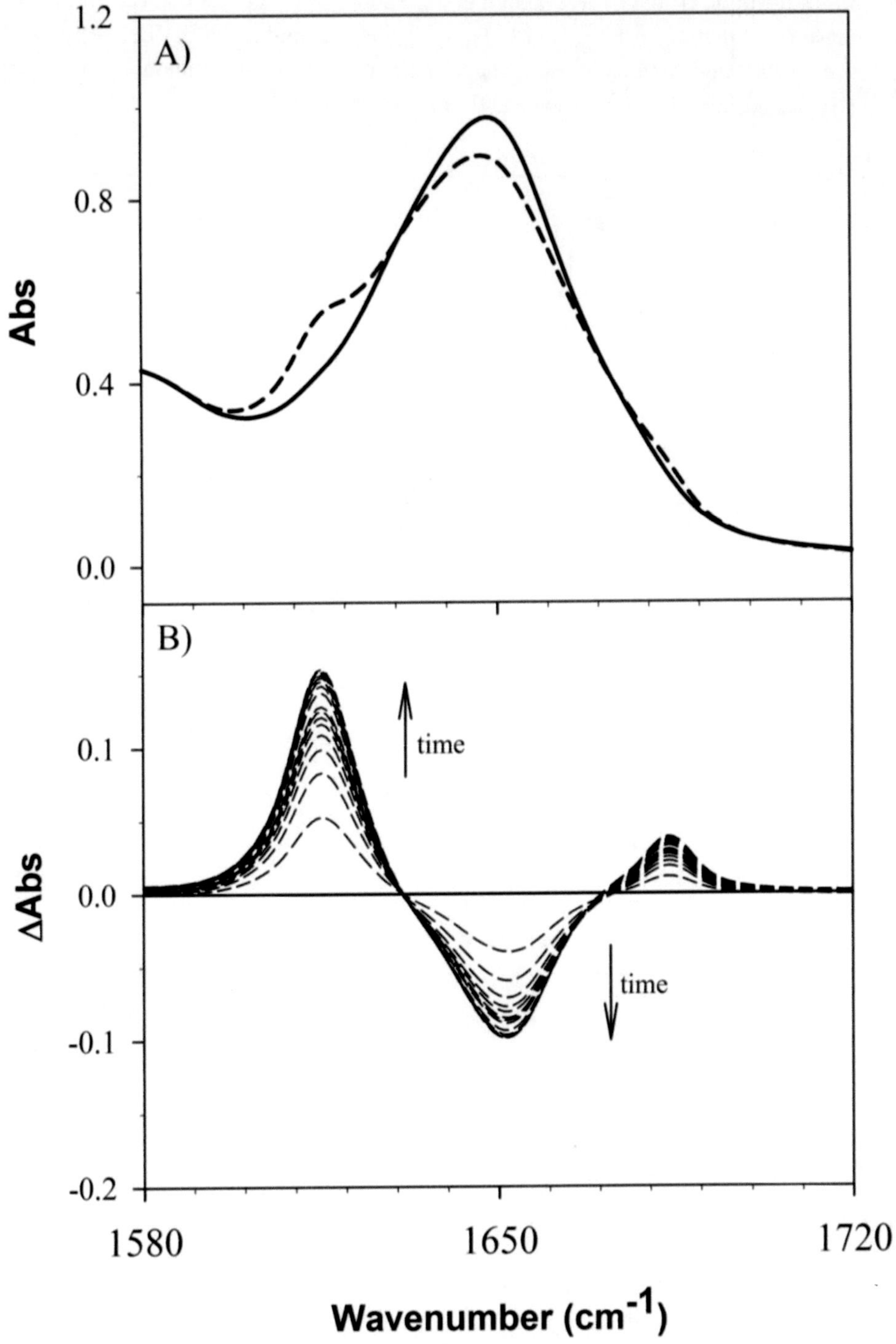

Figure 4. Panel (A): IR absorption spectra in the Amide I' region measured on a sample of 1mM BSA (pH = 7) at the initial (solid line) and final (dashed line) time of the incubation at T = 58 °C. Panel (B): IR absorption difference spectra recorded during the 2-hours incubation at T = 58 °C .

In particular, the absorption intensity at about 1,615 cm^{-1} is increased while the spectral component at about 1,650 cm^{-1} is decreased, indicating the conversion of α-helices into intermolecular β-sheets (Fang and Dalgleish, 1997; Qi et al., 1997; Fink, 1998; Allain et al., 1999; Lefevre and Subirade, 1999; Militello et al., 2003; Remondetto and Subirade, 2003). Figure 4B shows the complete time evolution of the absorption difference spectra. Note that the modifications induced in the secondary and tertiary structure of the protein by the thermal treatment are stable up to 8 hours. In Figure 5 we report the normalized light scattered intensity and the absorption difference at 1615 cm^{-1} and 1442 cm^{-1} as a function of time. The existence of a unique master curve suggests that, during the incubation at 58 °C, the partial BSA denaturation, the formation of aggregates and the secondary structural changes are all simultaneous events.

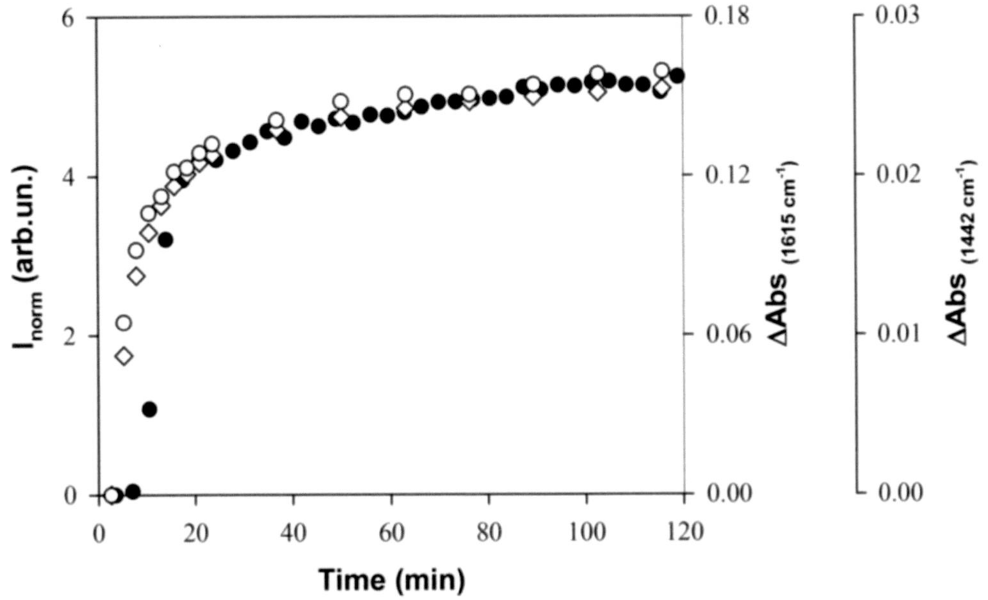

Figure 5. Comparison between the normalized light scattered intensity (black circles) and the differential absorbance of the Amide I' (empty diamonds) and Amide II' (empty circles) recorded at 1615 cm^{-1} and 1442 cm^{-1} respectively, during the 2-hours incubation at T = 58 °C of a sample of 1mM BSA (pH = 7).

To investigate the rheological properties of the protein solution after a 2-hour incubation, mechanical spectra have been measured. The results (not shown) indicate that the solution after the thermal treatment, presents a very weak elastic character with the elastic modulus slightly larger than the viscous one.

2.2. The Addition of Metal Ions as the Final Step of BSA Cold Gelation

Cold-gels of thermally treated BSA solution have been obtained after addition, at room temperature, of different concentration of $ZnCl_2$ and $CuCl_2$ salts. With the exclusion of the samples at the lowest salt concentration (1 mM in both cases) a marked solid-like character is observed a few minutes after the salt addition to the BSA solutions.

In Figure 6 the kinetic profiles of the elastic moduli (G') are reported for all concentrations of $ZnCl_2$ and $CuCl_2$ (panel A and B, respectively).

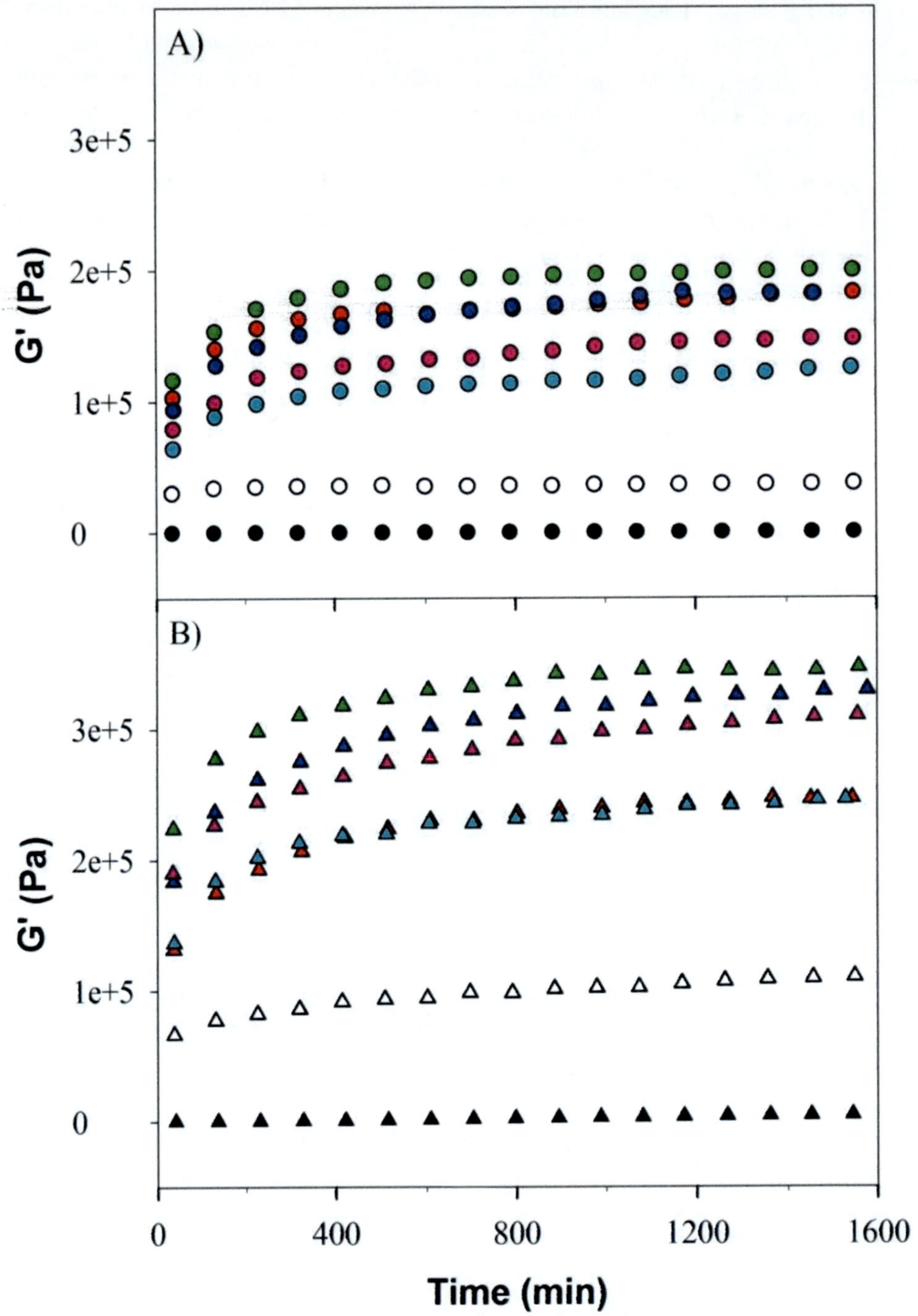

Figure 6. Rheological kinetic profiles at 1 rad/s of BSA gels obtained after addition of different amounts of $CuCl_2$ (panel A) or $ZnCl_2$ (panel B): 1 mM (black), 5 mM (white), 8 mM (red), 10 mM (green), 15 mM (blue), 20 mM (magenta) and 30 mM (cyan). The samples were put on the rheometry plate at T=20 °C after 2-hours incubation at T = 58 °C.

Figure 7 reports the elastic modulus value obtained at t=1500 minutes, as a function of ion concentration for the two ions studied. Data show that: i) Zn^{2+} has a stronger effect than Cu^{2+}, and ii) a maximum of the elastic modulus is observed at about 10 mM.

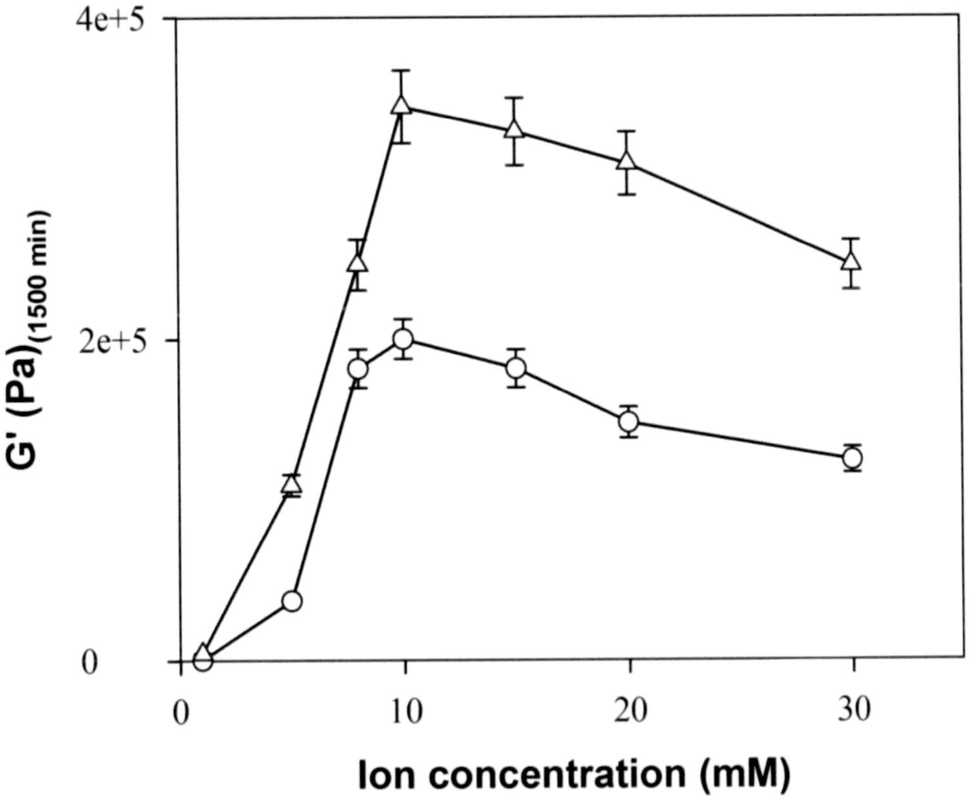

Figure 7.Dependence of the elastic modulus of BSA gels at T=20 °C and 1 rad/s, on the ion concentration: Cu^{2+} (circles), Zn^{2+} (triangles). The reported values were taken at 1500 minutes (see Figure 7).

Accordingly with the literature (Remondetto et al., 2002; Remondetto and Subirade, 2003; Marangoni et al., 2000) these results can be explained by considering that the gel supramolecular arrangement (Doi, 1993) changes as a function of the metal concentration. Below 10 mM salt concentration, at pH values far from isoelectric point, the negative charges present on the protein surface cannot be secluded. In this conditions an ordered assembly occurs in a "preferential" linear direction, and the network is formed by filamentous and fine structures. Gels so obtained are transparent, due to the small dimensions of the aggregated structures present in solution, and exhibit a large elastic value (Tobitani and Ross-Murphy, 1997). Above 10 mM salt concentration, the addition of large amount of ions in solution is capable of reducing the energy barrier preventing the molecular approaching. In these conditions, gels are made up by random and spherical connected aggregates ("particulate gels"). The network is coarse, opaque and brittle and characterized by a low elasticity. At intermediate protein/metal ratio, both filamentous and random structures are simultaneously present in the sample. Our results are in agreement with data obtained by Haque and Aryana (2002) for the thermal gelation of BSA. They found that the addition of 5 mM $ZnSO_4$ to BSA solutions causes the formation of a more compact and clustered gel compared with that obtained in presence of CuSO4. These results evidence the direct role of the metal ions in protein cold-gelation due to their capacity to act as bridges between the negative charged groups present on neighboring protein molecules (Ball et al. 1998; Bryant and McClements

1998; Navarra et al., 2007 and 2009a; Remondetto and Subirade 2003). Moreover, the higher G' value observed in presence of Zn^{2+} suggests that more sites are available on the protein surface for this ion making more frequent the links between different BSA molecules.

3. The Effects of Endogenous Ions: BSA Thermal Stability

The chromatographic separation of native BSA solution (hereafter reported as "not-treated BSA") (Figure 8) performed on a SEC-column, reveals the presence of BSA trimers, dimers and monomers (main peak) in the range 20–30 minutes in agreement with the literature data (Meyer, 2005).

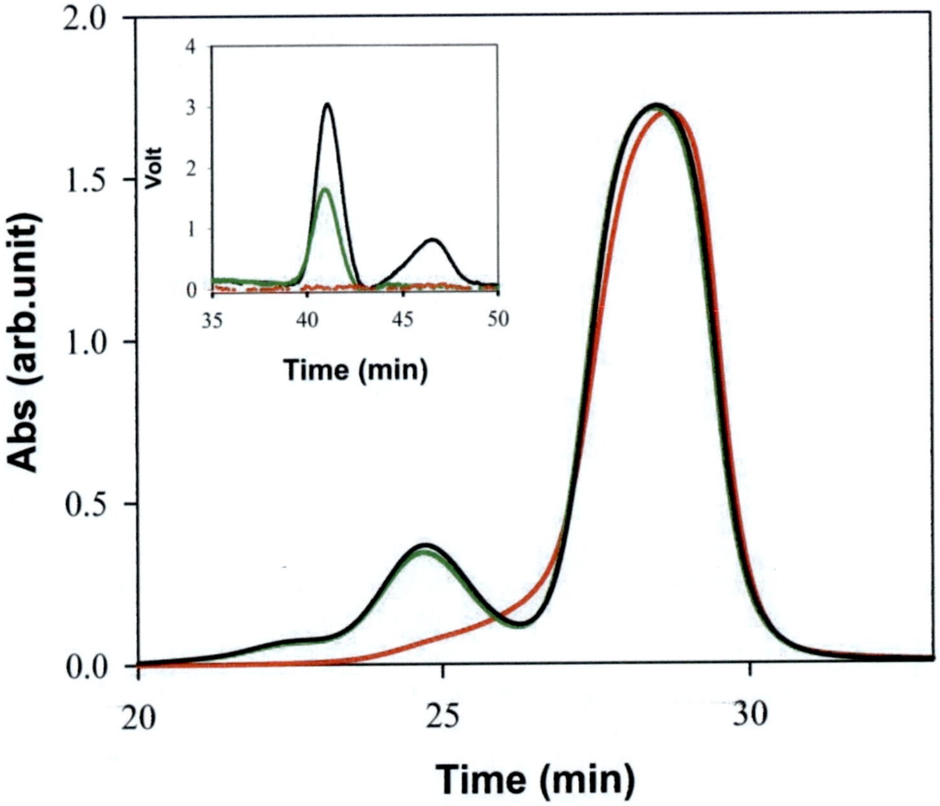

Figure 8. HPLC profiles at T = 20 °C of not-treated (black line), dialyzed (green line) and monomeric (red line) BSA samples (C = 0.15 mM). The inset shows the signal of the differential refractometer in line with the HPLC apparatus.

The signal of the differential refractometer, connected to the HPLC apparatus, showed two later small peaks, not detected by UV absorption. This could be assigned to the presence of salts in solution (Meyer, 2005) as often observed by using SEC-separation. When the collected monomeric fraction was re-injected in the SEC column, only a peak superimposed to the main one was obtained, indicating that the oligomeric species were not in equilibrium with the monomeric fraction. No changes were observed up to 24 hours. To investigate the chemical nature of the components responsible for the refractometric signal, a not-treated BSA solution was dialyzed for 24 hours and then injected in the HPLC. The signal perfectly overlapped with that of not-treated BSA within 30 min. elution, but some differences were present in the late part of the chromatogram, corresponding to the salt peaks (Figure 8, inset). This indicated that salts were only partially removed by dialysis. Inductively coupled plasma mass spectrometry (ICP-MS) analysis showed that main salt components were iron, copper and zinc ions strongly bound to the protein and not completely removed through dialysis process.

In order to investigate the role of these ions on the stability of the protein, fluorescence experiments were performed at room temperature. The emission spectra of monomeric BSA and not-treated BSA, excited at 270 nm, are shown in Figure 9.

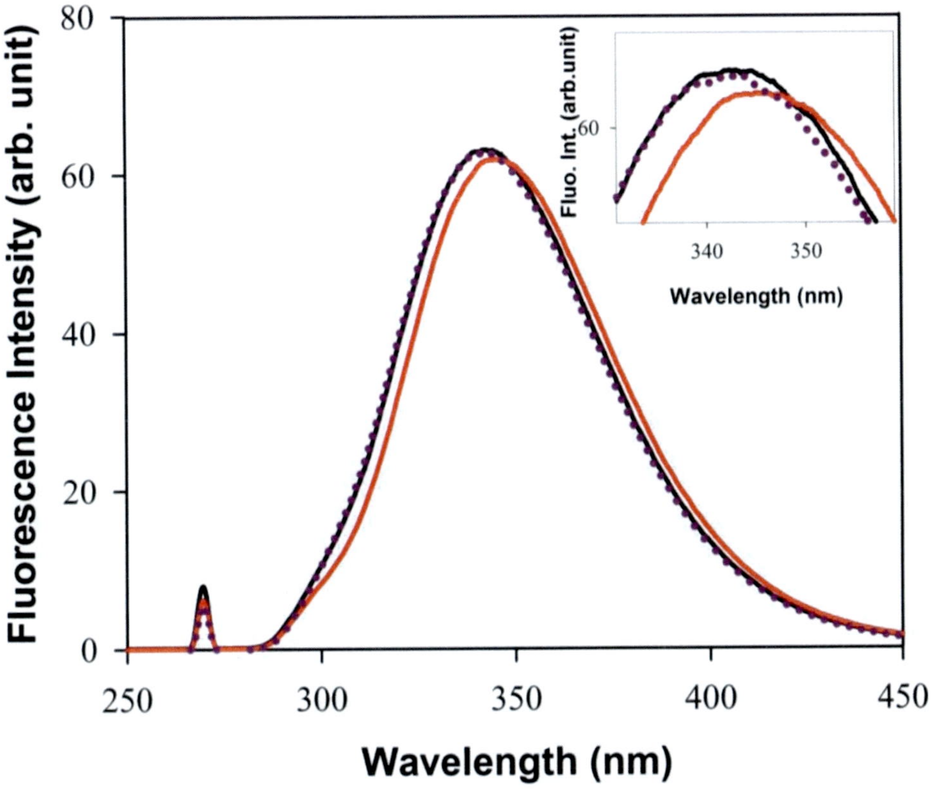

Figure 9. Fluorescence emission spectra at T = 20 °C of not-treated (black line), reconstituted (dotted violet line) and monomeric (red line) BSA samples (C = 0.015 mM). The inset shows the enlargement of the peak region.

A 3-nm red-shift is observed in case of monomeric BSA, indicating an increased exposure of fluorophore to the aqueous environment, that is a partial opening of the tertiary structure. If the initial proteinaceous and saline fractions, collected after HPLC separation, are mixed again (the sample is hereafter reported as "reconstituted BSA"), the fluorescence signal overlaps with that of not-treated BSA (see Figure 9) showing that the presence of ions in solution restores the native behaviour.

3. 1. The Thermal Stability of BSA Molecules

The effect of ions removal on BSA thermal stability was studied using temperature scanning and quenching experiments.

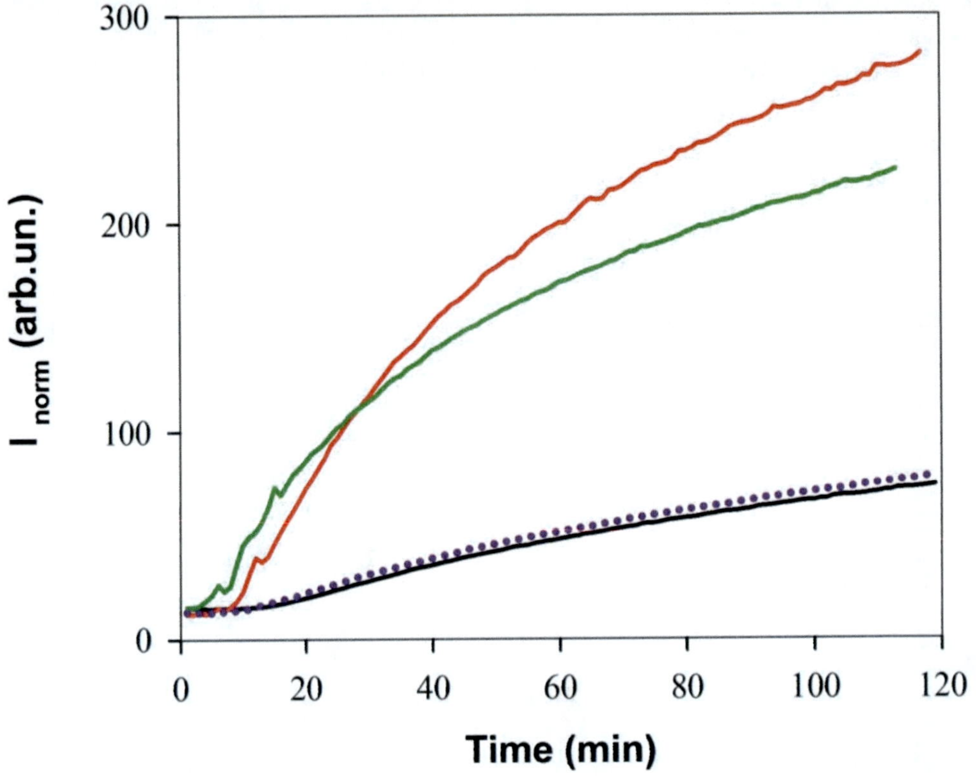

Figure 10. Normalized intensity growth of the scattered light as a function of time for not-treated (black line), reconstituted (dotted violet line), dialyzed (green line) and monomeric (red line) BSA samples (C = 0.03 mM, T = 67 °C).

Figure 10 reports the normalized light scattered intensity as a function of time, for not-treated, dialyzed, monomeric, and reconstituted BSA samples quenched at 67 °C. A higher growth rate of aggregates is observed when the ions are partially or totally removed, indicating that the protein is more prone to aggregation if deprived of endogenous ions and that the protein returns to the original behaviour, if all components are present in solution. As expected, the dyalized sample shows an intermediate profile if compared with not treated and monomeric samples.

Figure 11 shows results of Circular Dichroism and SLS temperature scanning experiments performed on the monomeric and not-treated BSA solutions. The sample deprived of ions is less thermally stable than the non-treated one since the aggregation process starts at lower temperature.

All together these results confirm that the monomeric BSA, devoided of its endogenous ions, is less compact and more prone to aggregation than the non-treated one.

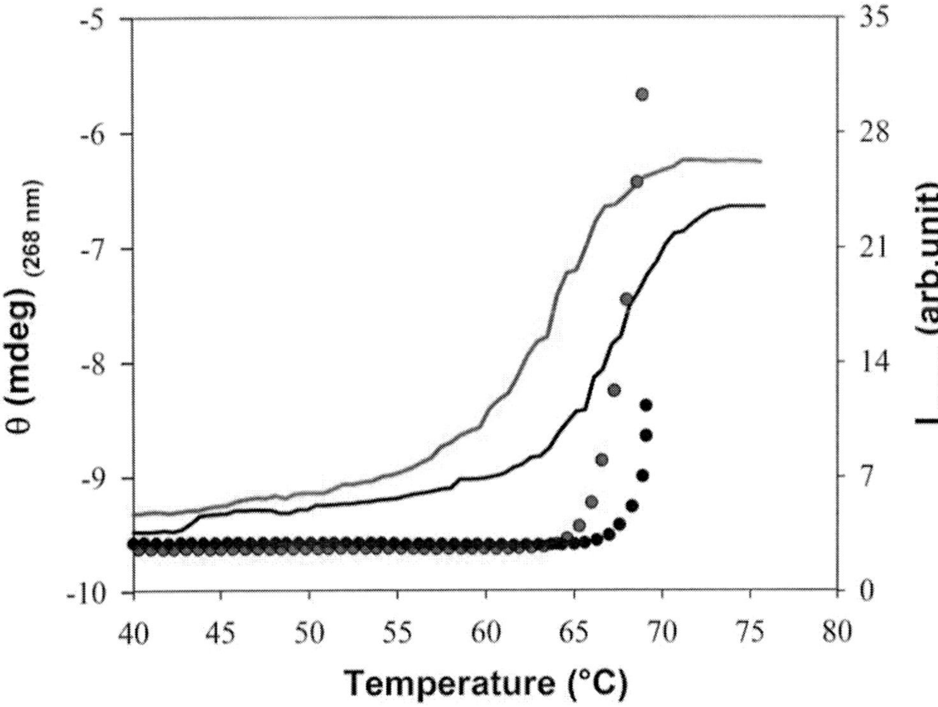

Figure 11. CD signal at 268 nm wavelength (line) and light scattered intensity (symbol) during the temperature scan experiments at a rate of 9°C/h on not-treated (black) and monomeric (red) samples of BSA (c = 3 μM).

4. Conclusion

Our results show that metal ions can play an opposite role on protein stability/aggregation. In fact, the addition of exogenous ions to solutions of BSA, thermally treated well below its denaturation threshold, leads to the formation of gels with a wide range of texture strength, depending on ion type and concentration. This procedure, named "cold gelation", has important applications in food or pharmaceutical technologies since it allows forming a strong gel at low temperature by preserving heat liable molecules.

On the other hand, the presence of endogenous ions, firmly bound to the protein, is important for its stability. Indeed, the removal of these ions by chromatographic separation causes a molecular structural change which, in turn, results in a higher aggregation rate under unfolding conditions.

5. Materials and Methods

5.1. Preparation of Cold-Gel Sample

Bovine serum albumin (Sigma Aldrich) was dissolved in 20 mM MES solution prepared either in H_2O or D_2O and titred with KOH or KDO to obtain a final pH or pD of 7 (where pD

= pH + 0.4). The final concentration of BSA was 1 mM. The protein solution was centrifuged for 8 minutes at 6100 g and filtered through Sartorius filters with pore size 0.2 μm. The samples containing D_2O were tested by IR and light scattering measurements. The D_2O was added to avoid the intense H20 band in the Amide I band region (1650 cm^{-1}). Stock solutions of $CuCl_2$ or $ZnCl_2$ (from Sigma Aldrich with a purity of 99.999%) were prepared in H_2O, and appropriate amounts were added to the protein solutions after the heating and cooling treatments.

5.2. Sample Preparation for HPLC Treatment

The protein was dissolved at the concentration of 0.3 mM in 50 mM phosphate buffer (pH 6.2). The solution was centrifuged at 6100 *g* for 10 min at 4°C and finally filtered through 0.2 μm filters.

The monomeric sample was obtained by injecting a 0.30 mM not-treated sample in a SEC-column and collecting the fraction corresponding to monomeric protein. The final monomeric sample concentration was obtained with the Amicon Ultracel 30 K concentrator.

An aliquot of the not-treated sample at the concentration 0.30 mM was dialyzed for 1 day in Spectra/Por membrane tubes, molecular weight cut-off 6000-8000, against phosphate buffer.

The reconstituted sample was obtained by mixing together the protein (trimers, dimers, and monomers) and salt fractions collected in the chromatographic experiment. The solution was therefore opportunely concentrated with Amicon Ultra- ultracel 30 K concentrators

5.3. IR Measurements

IR experiments were performed on a Bruker Vertex 70 Spectrophotometer, with a MIR global light source. Each spectrum was obtained by averaging over 100 scans. The spectral resolution was 2 cm^{-1}. The samples were placed between two CaF_2 windows, with a Teflon spacer of 0.05 mm. Each absorption spectrum was corrected for the contribution of the empty beam line and the residual water vapor spectrum. The error on the wavenumber was ± 1 cm^{-1} with absorbance accuracy within 1%.

Difference spectra were obtained by subtracting the spectrum recorded at the initial time from the spectrum taken at a generic *t* time. The initial spectrum was collected 7 minutes after the beginning of the experiments to allow the achievement of the thermal equilibrium. All experiments reported are the average of at least three measurements.

5.4. Static and Dynamic Light Scattering Measurements

Static and dynamic light scattering measurements were performed by using a Brookhaven Instrument BI-9000 digital correlator and a 200 mW solid state laser Ventus (laser quantum MPC 6000) tuned at a wavelength of 514.5 nm. Samples, prepared as described above, were put into a thermostatted cell holder of the Brookhaven Instrument BI200-SM goniometer system. Temperature was controlled within ± 0.1 °C using a thermostatted circulating bath. The normalized light scattered intensity was calculated as follows:

$$I_{norm} = (I_s - I_0)/(c * I_T)$$

where I_s, I_0 and I_T are the intensities of the light scattered by the sample, buffer and toluene, respectively, and c is the protein concentration in % (w/w).

Autocorrelation data were preliminarily analyzed using the cumulants method to obtain the mean size (Z- average diameter) of the particles present in solution. More detailed information on the size distribution of the species in solution was obtained by using CONTIN (Provencher, 1982).

DLS measurements were also performed by using a Zetasizer Nano – S90 (Malvern Instruments) equipped with a He-Ne laser source at a wavelength of 633 nm. Data were collected at 90°. The sample compartment was completely self-enclosed and its temperature was controlled within 0.1 °C.

5.5. Rheological Measurements

Rheological measurements were performed on a stress controlled AR 1000 rheometer (TA Instruments, USA) using a titanium-cone/plate geometry (angle 0.0174 rad, radius 20 mm, gap 26 μm). Viscoelastic spectra were done in the frequency range 0.1–200 rad/s, at a strain of 1×10^{-3} within the linear viscoelastic region.

The gelation kinetics of cold-gelling samples was obtained by viscoelastic spectra. The protein suspension, with the added salt, was gently stirred and placed on the rheometer plate, set at the temperature of 20 °C.

All measurements were done at least in triplicate.

5.6. HPLC Measurements

HPLC measurements were performed on a Shimadzu LC-2010 AT Prominence system equipped with a Degasser filter (DGU-$20A_5$), a 500 μl sample loop and an UV-VIS photodiode array detector (SPD-M20A). The HPLC apparatus was connected in line with a Brookhaven Instruments Co. differential refractometer A Superdex 200 10/300 GL SEC-column was used for analytical and preparative chromatographic experiments. The mobile phase was phosphate buffer at pH 6.2 (50 mM) pumped at 0.5 ml/min flow rate.

5.7. Circular Dichroism Measurements

Circular dichroism (CD) measurements were done by using a JASCO J-815 system. Near-UV signal at the wavelength of 268 nm was recorded by using a 0.2 cm optical path quartz cuvette. The protein concentration was 0.003 mM.

5.8. Fluorescence Measurements

Intrinsic fluorescence of solutions of BSA at concentration of 0.3 mM was measured on a JASCO FP-6500 spectrofluorimeter. The emission spectrum of the tryptophan was recorded in the range 250 – 450 nm with λ_{ex} = 270 nm. All measurements were performed at fixed gain.

ACKNOWLEDGMENTS

We thank Dr. Alessia Provenzano, Mr. Mario Lapis, Mr. Fulvio Ferrante for their technical support. A special thank to Dr. Sergio Bonomolo for the ICP-MS analysis.

REFERENCES

Allain, A.F., Paquin, P., Subirade, M. (1999) Relationships between conformation of β-lactoglobulin in solution and gel states as revealed by attenuated total reflection Fourier transform infrared spectroscopy. *Biol. Macromol.*, *26*, 337–344.

Alting A. (2003) A "cool" tool for industrial protein gelation. Nizo Food Research, 7 Available from: *www.nizo.com/files/19*

Alting, A.C., Weijers, M., de Hoog, E.H.A., van de Pijpekamo, A.M., Cohen Stuart, M.A., Hamer, R.J., de Kruif, C.G., Visschers, R.W. (2004) Acid induced cold gelation of globular proteins: effects of protein aggregate characteristics and disulfide bonding on rheological properties. *J. Agric. Food Chem.*, *52*, 623–631.

Bakker, J.M., Plutzer, C., Hunig, I., Haber, T,. Compagnon, I., von Helden, G., Meijer, G., Kleinermanns, K. (2005) Folding structures of isolated peptides as revealed by gas-phase mid-infrared spectroscopy. *Chem. Phys. Chem.*, *6*, 120

Ball, W., Christodoulou, J., Sadler, P.J., Tucker, A. (1998) Multi-metal binding site of serum albumin. *J. Inorg. Biochem.*, *70*, 33–39.

Barbut, S., Foegeding, E.A. (1993) Ca^{2+}-induced gelation of pre-heated whey protein isolate. *J. Food Sci.*, *58*, 867–871

Barreca, D., Laganà, G., Ficarra, S., Tellone, E., Leuzzi, U., Magazù, S., Galtieri, A., Bellocco, E. (2010) Anti-aggregation properities of trehalose on heat-induced secondary structure and conformation changes of bovine serum albumin. *Biophys. Chem.*, *147*, 146-152

Brange, J., Hallund, O., Sorensen, E. (1992) Chemical stability of insulin. 5. Isolation, characterization and identification of insulin transformation products. *Acta Pharm. Nord.*, *4*, 223-232

Brown, D.R. (2011) Prions and manganese: A maddening beast. *Metallomics*, *3*, 229-238

Bryant, C.M., McClements, D.J. (2000) Influence of NaCl and $CaCl_2$ on cold-set gelation of heat-denatured whey protein. *J. Food Sci.*, *65*, 801–804

Byler, D.M., Susi, H. (1986) Examination of the secondary structure of proteins by deconvolved FTIR spectra. *Biopolymers*, *25*, 469-487

Carter, D. C. and Ho, J. X. (1994) Serum Albumin. *Adv. Protein Chem.*, *45*, 153-203

Comai M., Dalla Serra M., Potrich C., Menestrina G. (2003) Cu^{2+} and Zn^{2+} effects on beta-amyloid aggregation and structural conformation. *Biophys. J.*, *84*, 337

Crichton R.R. (2008) Biological Inorganic Chemistry. An introduction. Elsevier

Curtain C.C., Ali F., Volitakis I., Cherny R.A., Norton R.S., Beyreuther K., Barrow C.J., Masters C.L., Bush A.I., Barnham K.J. (2001) Alzheimer's disease amyloid-beta binds copper and zinc to generate an allosterically ordered membrane-penetrating structure containing superoxide dismutase-like subunits. *J. Biol. Chem.*, *276*, 20466–20473

Davies P. D. Moualla and Brown D.R. (2011) Alpha-Synuclein is a cellular ferrireductase. *PLoS One*, *6*, e15814

Dobson M.C. (2004) Principles of protein folding, misfolding and aggregation. *Sem. Cell & Dev. Biol.*, *15*, 3-16

Doi E. (1993) Gels and gelling of globular proteins. *Trends Food Sci. Technol.*, *1*, 1–5.

Donaldson J. (1987) The physiopathologic significance of manganese in brain: its relation to schizophrenia and neurodegenerative disorders. *Neurotoxicology*, *8*, 451–462.

Dong, A., Huang, P., Caughey, W.S. (1990) Protein secondary structures in water from second-derivative Amide I infrared spectra. *Biochemistry*, *29*, 3303–3308

Fang, Y., Dalgleish, D.G. (1997) Conformation of ß-lactoglobulin studied by FTIR: effect of pH, temperature, and adsorption to the oil–water interface. *J. Colloid Interface Sci.*, *196*, 292–298

Fink, A.L. (1998) Protein aggregation: folding aggregates, inclusion bodies and amyloid. *Fold. Des.*, *30*, R9–R23

Fridovich, I. (1986) Superoxide dismutases. *Adv. Enzymol. Relat. Areas Mol. Biol.*, *58*, 61–97.

Gibson, T.D. (1996) Protein stabilisation using additives based on multiple electrostatic interactions. *Dev. Biol. Stand.*, *87*, 207–217

Haque, Z.Z. and Aryana, K.J. (2002) Effect of copper, iron, zinc and magnesium ions on bovine serum albumin gelation. *Food Sci. Technol. Res.*, *8*, 1-3

He, X.M. and Carter, D.C. (1992) Atomic structure and chemistry of human serum albumin. *Nature*, *358*, 209-215

Hirayama, K., Akashi, S., Furuya, M., Fukuhara, K. (1990) Rapid confirmation and revision of the primary structure of bovine serum albumin by ESIMS and frit-FAB LC/MS. *Biochem. Biophys. Res. Comm.*, *173*, 639-646

Hongsprabhas P., Barbut S. (1997) Ca^{2+}-induced cold gelation of whey protein isolate: effect of two stage gelation. *Food Res. Int.*, *30*, 523-527

Huang, B.X., Kim, H.Y., Dass, C. (2004). Probing three-dimensional structure of bovine serum albumin by chemical cross-linking and mass spectrometry. *J. Am. Soc. Mass Spectrom.*, *8*, 1237-47

Kavanagh, G.M., Clark, A.H., Ross-Murphy, B.S. (2000) Heat-induced gelation of globular proteins: part 3. Molecular studies on low pH b-lactoglobulin gels. *Int. J. Biol. Macromol.*, *28*, 41–50

Kawahara, M., Koyama, H., Nagata, T. and Sadakane, Y. (2011) Zinc, copper, and carnosine attenuate neurotoxicity of prion fragment PrP106-126. *Metallomics*, *330* DOI: 10.1039/C1MT00015B

Klug, A. (2010) The discovery of zinc fingers and their applications in gene regulation and genome manipulation. *Ann. Rev. Biochem.*, *79*, 213-231

Kosa, T., Maruyama, T., Otagiri, M. (1997) Species differences of serum albumins: I. Drug binding sites. *Pharm. Res.*, *14*, 1607–1612.

Kratochwil, N.A., Ivanov, A.I., Patriarca, M., Parkinson, J.A., Gouldsworthy, A.M., Murdoch, P.d.S., and Sadler, P.J. (1999) Surprising reactions of iodo Pt(IV) and Pt(II) complexes with Human Albumin: detection of Cys34 sulfenic acid. *J. Am. Chem. Soc.*, *121*, 8193-8203.

Lefevre, T., Subirade, M. (1999) Structural and interaction properties of ß -lactoglobulin as studied by FTIR spectroscopy. *Int. J. Food Sci. Technol.*, *34*, 419–428.

Lau, S.J., Sarkar, B. (1971) Ternary coordination complex between human serum albumin, copper (II), and L-histidine. *J. Biol. Chem.*, *246*, 5938-5943

Lu, J., Stewart, A.J., Sadler, P.J., Pinheiro, T.J.T., Blindauer, C.A. (2008) Albumin as a zinc carrier: properties of its high-affinity zinc-binding site. *Biochem Soc. Trans.*, *36*, 1317-1321

MacLean, D.S., Qiang, Q., Middaugh, C.R. (2002) Stabilization of proteins by low molecular weight multi-ions. *J. Pharm. Sci.*, *91*, 2220-2229

Marangoni, A.G., Barbut, S., McGauley, S.E., Marcone, M., Narine, S.S. (2000) On the structure of particulate gels - The case of salt induced cold gelation of heat-denatured whey protein isolate. *Food Hydrocoll.*, *14*, 61–74

Meyer, V. (2005) Practical high-performance liquid chromatography. J. Wiley & Sons

Militello, V., Vetri, V., Leone, M. (2003) Conformational changes involved in thermal aggregation processes of bovine serum albumin. *Biophys. Chem.*, *105*, 133–141.

Navarra, G., Giacomazza, D., Leone, M., Librizzi, F., Militello, V., San Biagio, P.L. (2009a) Thermal aggregation and ion-induced cold-gelation of bovine serum albumin. *Eur. Biophys. J.*, *38*, 437-446

Navarra, G., Leone, M., Militello, V. (2007) Thermal aggregation of ß lactoglobulin in presence of metal ions. *Biophys. Chem.*, *161*, 52–61.

Navarra, G., Tinti, A., Leone, M., Militello, V., Torreggiani, A (2009b) Influence of metal ions on thermal aggregation of bovine serum albumin: aggregation kinetics and structural changes. *J. Inorg. Biochem.*, *103*, 1729-1738

Ostojic, S., Dragutinovic, V., Kicanovic, M., Simonovic, B.R. (2007) A DSC study of zinc binding to bovine serum albumin (BSA) *J. Serb. Chem. Soc.*, *72*, 331-337

Peters, Jr. T. (1995) All about Albumin: biochemistry, genetics and medical applications. Academic Press, New York.

Provencher, S.W. (1982) CONTIN: A general purpose constrained regularization program for inverting noisy linear algebraic and integral equations. *Comput. Phys. Commun.*, *27*, 229-242

Qi, X.L., Holt, C., McNulty, D., Clarke, D.T., Brownlow, S., Gareth R., Jones G.R. (1997) Effect of temperature on the secondary structure of b-lactoglobulin at pH 6.7, as determined by CD and IR spectroscopy: a test of the molten globule hypothesis. *Biochem. J.*, *324*, 341–346

Ragoonanan, V. and Aksan, A. (2007) Protein stabilization. *Transfus. Med. Hemother.*, *34*, 246-252

Rasia, R.M., Bertoncini, C.W., Marsh, D., Hoyer, W., Cherny, D., Zweckstetter, M., Griesinger, C., Jovin, T.M. and Fernandez, C.O. (2005) Structural characterization of copper(II) binding to α-synuclein: Insights into the bioinorganic chemistry of Parkinson's disease. *Proc. Natl. Acad. Sci. USA.*, *102*, 4294–4299

Ratnaparkhi, G.S. and Varadarajan R. (2001) Osmolytes stabilize ribonuclease S by stabilizing its fragments S protein and S peptide to compact folding-competent states. *J. Biol. Chem.*, *276*, 28789-28798

Remondetto, G.E., Paquin, P., Subirade, M. (2002) Cold gelation of b-lactoglobulin in the presence of iron. *J. Food Sci.*, *67*, 586-595

Remondetto, G.E., Subirade, M. (2003) Molecular mechanism of Fe^{2+} induced ß - lactoglobulin cold gelation. *Biopolymers*, *69*, 461-469

Rosen, D.R, Siddique, T., Patterson, D., Figlewicz, D.A., Sapp, P., Hentati, A., Donaldson, D., Goto, J., O'Regan, J.P., Deng, H.X, Rahmani, Z., Krizus, A., McKenna-Yasek, D., Cayabyab, A., Gaston, S.M., Berger, R., Tanzi, R.E., Halperin, J.J., Herzfeldt, B., Van den Bergh, R., Hung, W.-Y., Bird, T., Deng, G., Mulder, D. W., Smith, C., Laimg, N.G., Soriano, E., Pericak-Vance, M.A., Haines, J., Smyth, G.A., Gusella, J.S., Horvitz, H.R. and Brown, R.H. Jr. (1993) Mutations in Cu/Zn superoxide dismutase gene are associated with familial amyotrophic lateral sclerosis. *Nature*, *362*, 59–62.

Ryall, R.J. (1974) Competitive dialysis studies of metal-protein equilibria. Australian National University, Canberra

Sarkar, B., Wigfield, Y. (1968) Evidence for Albumin-Cu(II)-Amino Acid Ternary Complex. *Can. J. Biochem.*, *46*, 601-607

Stewart, A.J., Blindauer, C.A., Berezenko, S., Sleep, D., Sadler, P.J. (2003) Interdomain zinc site on human albumin. *Proc. Natl. Acad. Sci. USA*, *100*, 3701-3706

Surewicz, W.K., Mantsch, H.H. (1988) New insight into protein secondary structure from resolution-enhanced infrared spectra. *Biochim. Biophys. Acta*, *29*, 115-130

Tanzi, R.E., Petrukhin, K., Chernov, I., Pellequer, J.L. , Wasco, W., Ross, B., Romano, D.M., Parano, E., Pavone, L. and Brzustowicz, L.M., et al. (1993) The Wilson disease gene is a copper transporting ATPase with homology to the Menkes disease gene. *Nat. Genet.*, *5*, 344–350.

Theunissen, O., Rudt, F., Guddat, U., Mentzel, H., Pieler, T. (1992) RNA and DNA binding zinc fingers in Xenopus TFIIIA. *Cell*, *71*, 679-90

Tobitani, A., Ross-Murphy, S.B. (1997) Heat-induced gelation of globular proteins. 1. Model for the effects of time and temperature on the gelation time of BSA gels. *Macromolecules*, 30, 4845-4854.

Tougu, V., Tilman, A., Palumaa, P. (2011) Interactions of Zn(II) and Cu(II) ions with Alzheimer's amyloid-beta peptide. Metal ion binding, contribution to fibrillization and toxicity. *Metallomics*, *3*, 250-261

Volpe, S.L. , Lowe, N.M., Woodhouse, L.R. and King, J.C. (2007) Effect of maximal exercise on the short-term kinetics of zinc metabolism in sedentary man. *Br. J. Sports Med.*, *41*, 156-161.

Vulpe, C., Levinson, B., Whitney, S., Packman, S. and Gitschier, J. (1993) Isolation of a candidate gene for Menkes disease and evidence that it encodes a copper-transporting TPase. *Nat. Genet.*, *3*, 7–13.

Weijers, R.N.M. (1977) Amino acid sequence in bovine serum albumin. *Clin. Chem.*, *23*, 1361-1362

Xu, X., Zhang, L., Shen, D., Wu, H., Liu, Q. (2008) Oxygen-dependent oxidation of Fe(II) to Fe(III) and interaction of Fe(III) with Bovine Serum Albumin, leading to a hysteretic effect on the fluorescence of Bovine Serum Albumin. *J. Fluoresc.*, *18*, 193-201

INDEX

A

B

C

D

H

I

N

O

P

Q

R

S

T

U

V

W

X

Y

Z